Praise for Ly

Hope for Famil
with Congenit;

"A wonderful combination of practical information, moral support, and spiritual guidance."

~ Carlen Gomez-Fifer, MD
Associate Professor, Pediatric Cardiology
University of Michigan, C.S. Mott Children's Hospital

"This is a much-needed book caring for the whole family of children with serious heart and other medical conditions."

~ Dr. Stephen Beasley, Pediatric Emergency Physician,
TC Thompson Children's Hospital, Chattanooga, TN

"Each year more than 40,000 children and adolescents are diagnosed with congenital heart defects. If you are a parent who has a child with CHD, this book is for you. You need not walk alone. Lynda Young brings you the benefit of hearing the voices of others who have walked this road. It is truly a book of Hope."

~ Gary Chapman, Ph.D.
Author, *The Five Love Languages* and *Love As a Way of Life*

"This book is like a good recipe for living life, sprinkling CHD parents with hope, encouragement and comfort to continue their journey in being the best parents they can be."

~ Kathy Murphy, M.S.N., R.N., C.S.
Clinical Nurse Specialist
Children's Healthcare of Atlanta-Egleston
Sibley Heart Center

"This book is a GPS for the mind, body, and soul of families dealing with a child suffering from a congenital heart defect. It's filled with survival tools, inspiring stories, and life-saving advice. Most of all, you'll know you are not alone on a journey you didn't expect."

~ Carol Kent, Speaker and Author
When I Lay My Isaac Down (NavPress)

H♥pe

for Families of Children with Congenital Heart Defects

YOU are NOT ALONE Book Series

H❤pe

for Families of Children
with Congenital Heart Defects

Lynda T. Young

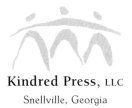

Kindred Press, LLC
Snellville, Georgia

Hope for Families of Children with Congenital Heart Defects
by Lynda T. Young;
The YOU are NOT ALONE Book Series

Published by Kindred Press, LLC
a division of Kindred Spirits International, P.O. Box 360666, Snellville, Georgia 30039

This book is available in volume at discount for qualifying organizations, such as churches, hospitals, and associations, and bookstores. Please contact the publisher to inquire: www.kindredpress.com

For more information about this book or The YOU are NOT ALONE Book Series, please visit www.HopeForFamiliesOnline.com

Cover and interior design by Another Jones Design

Publisher's Cataloging-In-Publication Data
(Prepared by The Donohue Group, Inc.)

Young, Lynda T.
   Hope for families of children with congenital heart defects / Lynda T. Young.

   p. ; cm. -- (YOU are NOT ALONE book series)

   Includes bibliographical references and index.
   ISBN: 978-0-9797800-2-8

   1. Congenital heart disease in children--Popular works. 2. Congenital heart disease in children--Psychological aspects--Family relationships--Popular works. 3. Congenital heart disease in children--Patients--Family relationships--Popular works. I. Title.

RJ426.C64 Y68 2010
362.1/9/612/043/3

Printed in the United States of America

Dedication

For my grandmother, Lizzy Tinnin, who, from her blue over-stuffed chair, loved the Lord, and the rest of us, with her whole heart. Heart disease took her dream of being a missionary and sharing Jesus in China, but that desire would be played out through her family's life instead.

"She made Jesus and the Bible come alive for us three children as we sat at her feet, enthralled at her stories. All of us grew up and served Him in places she never saw," my dad said.

Grandma Tinnin always had a smile, crocheting bedspreads and tablecloths for the family — while sharing words of encouragement with us grandchildren — she made me think I was the best at whatever I did. I knew that if no one else in the world was praying for me — she was.

With the physical challenges that confined her to home, some might say hers was a wasted life — but her love for Jesus and others spread from that blue chair all around the world. *Her damaged heart kept her from traveling in that world, but He reached it through her and the legacy of love that she left for all of us to share.*

Acknowledgments

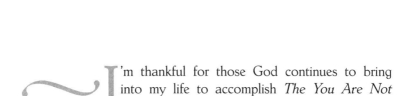

I'm thankful for those God continues to bring into my life to accomplish *The You Are Not Alone Book Series*. It's a team effort from many states and countries.

To the families, children and medical staff who've shared their heart journey, and bring hope to others. Peer review's helpful insights are woven into the final book.

To Sharon Castlen, *Integrated Book Marketing*, New York. Lisa Kay Hauser, book editing, Wisconsin. Anita Jones, *Another Jones Graphics*, Oregon. Mickey O'Brien, *Completely Coachable*, California.

To people who prayed through the writing of this book and prayed for those who will read it—you know who you are, and so does He.

To my husband John, who gives me total support and encouragement—and for overlooking computers, papers, books, and files piled high on the kitchen table.

And most importantly, to the One our hope is in.

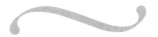

Foreword

Foreword from a Heart Mom

My name is Colleen and I am a mom of a child with a CHD, therefore, I'm a 'Heart Mom.' Actually, I'm a mom of two children with CHDs...and another with a 'healthy heart.'

I've learned many things on this heart journey, and one thing I've realized is that regardless of what's happening, anything involving your child is a big deal to you. Whether it's ear tubes, severe CHDs, mild CHDs...anything — even a broken bone that you know will soon heal. When your child hurts, you hurt. Your concerns, worries, and fears are valid.

Our oldest child, Matthew, was born with a 'healthy heart,' but he had a collapsed lung at birth and spent his first six days of life in the special care nursery. We were first time parents and initially terrified at this unexpected news. After our short 'ordeal,' we took him home and he thrived. At fourteen months, after several ear infections, his doctor told us that he would need minor surgery to place tubes in his ears. Minor surgery? It was our child and I thought, how could any surgery be 'minor?' We got through it and all was well.

Next came our second child, Tommy. At my twenty week ultrasound we were given devastating news, "Your baby has a severe Congenital Heart Defect called Hypoplastic Left Heart Syndrome (HLHS)." Our options were explained: termination of the pregnancy, multiple open heart surgeries, or 'compassionate care' after birth. Suddenly, perspective took place when recalling our older son's ear surgery.

Our third child, Genevieve, was thankfully diagnosed with a 'healthy heart' *in utero*. However, at age three a heart murmur was detected, and her pediatrician told us, "She has a less severe CHD, which will hopefully never need intervention, but we will follow it." Because we were already walking this heart journey with Tommy, again we were able to put the news in perspective.

I've come to realize, after being on this CHD road for ten years, that no one really gets how this road gets to you — except God. I find that when I pause and pour my heart out to HIM, even my frustrations with others not getting it, along with my own fears of what could happen to my child — that's when I receive the most comfort and peace. We are simply not in control of what happens to us or our children, even though we are their parents. They are truly 'on loan' to us and we must take one day at a time knowing how blessed we are to be chosen as their parents.

Lynda Young has blessed us with this book of real stories, helpful hints and most of all, HOPE. This book would have been helpful for our family in the early years of our journey, and I hope that it helps make your road just a little bit easier to travel.

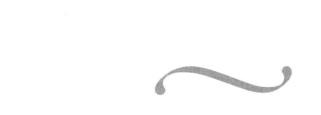

Contents

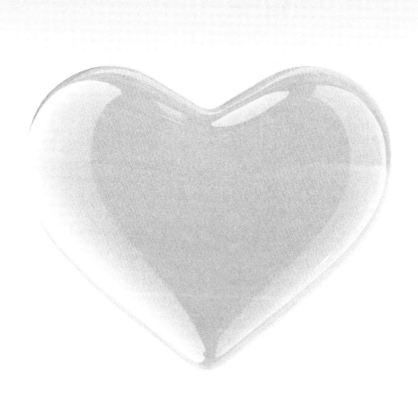

Hope...

"What floor do you want?"

It was noon at the children's hospital. Four weary-looking families wearing fluorescent lime-green "Visitor" name tags crowded around the closed elevator doors. One dad rolled his shoulders back to work the kinks out of his neck and glanced at the blinking green of the descending numbers — six, stop...five, stop...four, stop...three, stop...two, stop...one — doors opened, and people poured out. The families edged their way into the crowded car. Parents maneuvered IV poles and pushed two children sitting in small wheelchairs. Doors slowly shut.

"You can always tell when it's lunch time, can't you?" a dad asked.

Everyone nodded and smiled. "Okay, what floor do you want?"

People spoke numbers, he pushed buttons. "Everyone have a good day," and with his cheerful greeting, all smiles broadened.

Different floors, different diagnoses, different stories. Second floor — heart, third — cancer, fourth — kidney, fifth — many other diagnoses, and sixth — same day surgery. Each room on each floor held a story of a child and a family, many feeling alone and scared. But for a brief time — all responded to heart-felt encouraging words and a smile.

The *YOU are NOT ALONE Book Series* began with *Hope for Families of Children with Cancer*, and now continues with *Hope for Families of Children with Congenital Heart Defects*. Many challenges and issues are similar in both books. The same, but different. All need to experience rays of hope no matter what their story.

After you finish this book, look to the resources in the back for Inspiring Reading and Websites & Organizations to help you continue your journey.

So, what floor do *you* want? If you are a heart family, your 'extended' heart family is here for you. We come alongside you and your family in this book to share our experiences and encouraging words — *you are not alone*.

Blessings, Lynda

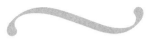

What's a CHD?

You passed me in the shopping mall
(You read my faded tee)
You tapped me on the shoulder
Then asked, "What's a CHD?"

I could quote terminology
There's stats that I could give
But I would rather share with you
A mother's perspective.

What is it like to have a child with a CHD?

It's Lasix, aspirin, Captopril
It's wondering...Lord, what's your will?
It's monitors and oxygen tanks
It's a constant reminder to always give thanks
It's feeding tubes, calories, needed weight gain
It's the drama of eating — and yes, it's insane!

It's the first time I held him (I'd waited so long)
It's knowing that I need to help him grow strong
It's making a hospital home for awhile
It's seeing my reward in every smile.

It's checking his stats as the feeding pump's beeping
It's knowing that there is just no time for sleeping
It's caths, x-rays, and boo boos to kiss
It's normalcy that sometimes I miss
It's asking, "Do his nails look blue?"
It's cringing inside at what he's been through.

It's dozens of calls to his pediatrician
(She knows me by name. I'm a mom on a mission)
It's winter's homebound and hand sanitizer
It's knowing this journey has made me much wiser
It's watching him sleeping — his breathing is steady
It's surgery day and I'll never be ready.

It's handing him over (I'm still not prepared)
It's knowing that his heart must be repaired
It's waiting for news on that long stressful day
It's praying, it's hoping that he'll be okay.

It's the wonderful friends with whom I've connected
It's the bond that we share, it was so unexpected
It's that long faded scar down my child's small chest
It's touching it gently and knowing we're blessed
It's watching him chasing a small butterfly
It's the moment I realized I've stopped asking, "Why?"
It's the snowflakes that fall on a cold winter's day
(They remind me of those who aren't with us today)
It's a brave little boy who loved Thomas the Train
Or a special heart bear or a frog in the rain
It's the need to remember we are all in this plight
It's their lives that remind us we still need to fight!
It's in pushing ahead amidst every sorrow
It's finding the strength to have hope for tomorrow.

And no, we'll never be the same
It's changed our family
This is what we face each day
This is a CHD.

— *Stephanie Husted, Heart Mom*

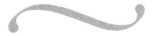

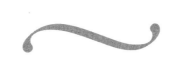

What comes from the heart goes to the heart.

~ **Samuel Taylor Coleridge**

Chapter One

Carved Initials

"Years ago, I let her know I loved her by carving our initials in the bark of an old tree in the woods near her house," an eighty-year-old husband said. "Then to be sure she understood my intentions, I carved a heart around them."

Initials, hearts, and love fill your world too. Initials may include CHD, VSD, HLHS — but all have your heart carved around them.

In this book, you're joined by those who've come alongside you on this journey. They are families of the heart.

One Size Does Not Fit All

This book is for the parent/family member/friend/medical professionals of any child born with a Congenital Heart Defect (CHD). There's a broad spectrum of CHDs: some less severe which require no intervention, some one-time intervention, and others a lifetime of intervention. Parts of this book will apply to your journey, and other parts may not. Either way, when you read this book, we hope you'll have a fuller understanding of the CHD journey. Wherever you are on this road, we want you to know that *you are not alone*.

Incidence of Congenital Heart Defects (Disease)

Most people are unaware that up to 1.3 million Americans alive today have some form of congenital heart defect and about one-half of these individuals are less than 25 years of age.

"I never knew babies could have heart disease," a heart mom said. "And, I assumed a baby died if she had one," another one added.

"When I heard 'disease' I assumed it was contagious."

All these assumptions are false, but are typical unless you've known someone on this CHD journey.

At least nine of every 1,000 infants born a year have a heart defect. That's almost one percent of live-born infants. Sometimes the defect is so mild that there are no outward symptoms. In other cases, it's so severe that the newborn becomes ill soon after birth. In still other cases, signs and symptoms occur only later in childhood.

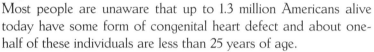

Helps & Hope

Initials — Some on the heart journey

CHD
Congenital Heart Defects or Congenital Heart Disease

VSD
Ventricular Septal Defect

HLHS
Hypoplastic Left Heart Syndrome

Helps & Hope

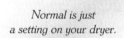

Normal is just a setting on your dryer.

— Patsy Clairmont

In the United States, about 40,000 children are born with a heart defect each year. Most of these children can be helped by surgery even if the defect is severe. There is hope.

Your "New Normal"

"So, how are you doing?"

Only those who've traveled this heart journey will understand your *new normal*. When others ask, "So, how are you doing?" they truly care, but some just can't or don't want to open themselves to your pain — especially if they have children with healthy hearts.

"When I heard about Amy's baby with a heart defect, I just pictured my baby being whisked away in the helicopter," said a new mom. "I'd never be able to handle that."

How *do* you answer the question? Smile, thank them for their concern, have a brief answer prepared, and ask for their prayers.

"Now, just what is wrong with your child's heart?"

You want to give them a bottom line answer because they probably won't understand — and you may not either at the beginning. Write out a two sentence diagnosis that you can tell them without thinking. The professionals or other heart parents can help you with this. If the questioner's eyes divert over your shoulder, or glaze over, then stop. You will find out quickly who can take in more and who can't. A prepared answer will

Helps & Hope

New Care Words used in the book

Words from the world of pediatric heart defects — the new normal:

HK
Heart Kid

HH
Healthy Heart (usually a sibling)

Caregiver
Person(s) giving care to the HK
(usually family members)

Coming-along-siders
Family, friends, and medical staff
who encourage HKs, HHs, and
their caregivers

help you when all the new heart jargon whirls in your mind — your new normal.

Connections
There are levels of friendship. Some people you know for years but share only the surface of life. With others, you share more and go deeper. But then there are those with whom you share a crisis — and you dive deep fast.

In this book, parents from all over the country (and overseas) share their stories and connect through their universal crisis: childhood heart defects. They've shared their journeys with us in this book hoping to connect and come alongside you, the reader. Some of the stories are compilations of several similar experiences.

I haven't walked this difficult path, but I am privileged to share these journeys with you.

On your journey, keep your eyes open for those with whom you'll share struggles, deep valleys, and God's provisions. Don't miss these opportunities; and more importantly, don't miss Him. *You're not alone.*

*Come to Me, all [you], who labor, and are
heavy laden, and I will give you rest.*
Matthew 11:28

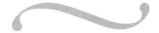

I believe in the sun even when it is not shining.
I believe in love even when I feel it not.
I believe in God even when He is silent.

— Words found written on a cellar wall in Cologne
after World War II

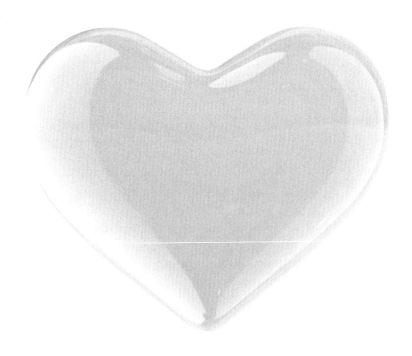

Chapter Two

I'm Sorry to Tell You This....

"This is the last thing we ever expected. Our baby has a heart problem?" We wonder how many disbelieving parents have said those words.

"She's only a baby. You just don't expect children to have heart problems. That's for old people."

However, each year more than 40,000 children and adolescents are diagnosed with congenital heart defects (CHDs) in the United States. This may seem like a small percentage compared to the millions of children twenty and younger in the United States, but not to parents walking this path with their child.

"What do you mean 'a small percentage'?" Jacob said as he reeled from his daughter's heart diagnosis. "The percentage doesn't matter when it's your child. I've never felt so helpless or alone. Obviously, those people have never had a critically ill child."

Helpless, alone, overwhelmed. All are normal feelings — you aren't losing your mind — it just feels that way. Many heart families label this the *new normal* as their lives adjust to new people, new places, and new protocols.

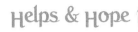

Helps & Hope

It's Okay...

It's okay to cry — tears clear our vision. Dads, that's for you too.

A New Room

"A nurse took my baby from me, and the cardiologist on duty said, 'Someone take the parents to the *Quiet Room*.' He said someone would be in to talk to us shortly. We sat there alone in that little room — where there were nothing but tissues and a telephone on the table — and waited. Then the chaplain walked in, and our hearts stopped — something had to be really wrong."

When you hear, "I'm sorry to tell you this, your child has a heart defect," your life splits into two parts: life before this information, and life with it. Each day demands new decisions, presents new challenges, and draws out perseverance that you never knew you had. Each day may bring you to the point of exhaustion, and still you keep going.

"But you'll also experience kindness from the hospital staff — a nurse played lullabies in the ICU to calm our baby (and us parents) — a medical tech brought an armload of blankets so we could make a pallet on the floor for my husband (since I occupied the only sleeper chair) — and there was even a smile from the lady who cleaned our hospital room floor," a mom said.

Whether you've just begun this journey, or persisted for weeks, months, or years, we want to encourage you with stories from your fellow travelers. Others have gone before you and, unfortunately, others will follow. Every CHD story is unique, but all share similar

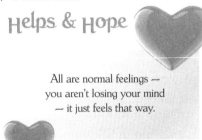

Helps & Hope

All are normal feelings — you aren't losing your mind — it just feels that way.

struggles, trials, and hopes. As a heart family, your life has been split in two parts. This book brings hope for that second part. **You are not alone.**

When the Wright family approached that second part, a heart defect was the last thing they ever expected.

One Family's Story
Before the Diagnosis: Approaching the Tunnel

"I'm marrying 'Mr. Right,'" Allison told her high school English students. "Of course his name is W-R-I-G-H-T, but he's certainly my Mr. Right."

And so began the fairy tale. Allison and Jason were married, moved into a two-story house, and had their first son, Caleb. Allison loved being a stay-at-home mom, cooked delicious meals, and adored her family — while Jason succeeded in his sales career. The fairy tale continued as they invited neighbors for meals, Bible studies, and times to sit around their fireplace and talk.

"We'd planned on more children, and were thrilled when I was pregnant with our second son. The pregnancy went smoothly, and because Caleb had been healthy, we assumed the next one would be also. As my tummy grew, we spent hours painting the baby's walls red and blue, and pasting the train border around the top of those walls. Now we were ready."

The Diagnosis: Sucked into Darkness

Allison's parents were visiting when she said, "I think it's time." Jason grabbed her suitcase, and they kissed Caleb goodbye. "We're going to the hospital to have baby Nathan." The only concern they had was the adjustment of first-born to the second-born.

Nathan's birth was an easy delivery, but he was a little bit blue. The 'baby team' suctioned him, pinked him up, and the nurse said he was perfectly healthy.

"The next morning, our Pediatrician came in to congratulate us and meet her newest patient. She told us, 'There's a heart murmur, but it's probably nothing to worry about, it's quite common. We're going to do some tests just to be on the safe side.' A little later, a white-coat lady came in and said, 'I'm here to take him for his tests' — and then she left. I was all by myself and didn't have a clue what was going on. I kept watching the clock on the wall — one hour went by, then two...and as difficult as it was to walk, I paced the halls and told the hospital staff, 'I want my baby now. What's going on?'

'He's fine in the NICU (neonatal intensive care unit),' was the only answer I got. Then, 'A doctor will be in later and let you know what's going on.'"

"Later, we did find out what was going on — and it was devastating. 'Your son has a very serious heart defect and will need surgery,' the doctor in the white coat told us.

"Are you saying he's going to die? A *major* defect?" Allison said.

"The pediatric cardiologist clinically explained what the plan would be — weekly doctor visits, future surgeries, medical terms thrown at me that made no sense — and she ended with, 'Take him home and just live normally.'"

Is she kidding?

"What do you mean 'normally'?"

"Treat him like any other baby," was the doctor's calm reply.

"As crazy as that sounded, it was good advice. I was to change his diaper, feed him, and do the *normal* things you do with a baby — the basics."

The doctor continued, "And bring him in if he starts to have trouble breathing, or if his gums, lips, or nail beds turn blue."

"Your other children and other people's kids are your frame of reference — normal things — but it seems like there's no frame of reference for a baby with a major heart defect. Heart surgery is for old people with bypasses, not for my baby — all that kept bombarding my mind," Allison said.

So they took one-week-old Nathan home to live a *normal* life. The red and blue room with trains on the border, trains painted on the bed, and toy trains placed on the dresser belied the fact that everything was normal. "I sat in my wooden rocking chair, cuddling this perfect-looking baby — wondering, *how am I going to know if something is wrong?* I asked everyone, 'Do his nails look blue?'"

They took him every few days for checkups and he was fine —

until one day — they heard the dreaded words. "He's in heart distress and we need to get him to the hospital for a heart cath."

It was Friday afternoon, and surgeries weren't scheduled on the weekend. In the meantime, the nurses carefully worked on Nathan to keep him comfortable. Suddenly, though, things took a turn for the worse and the nurse hit the dreaded button: Code Blue.

"All the air was sucked out of the room as people ran in with crash carts — they seemed to run out of the walls and filled up that small space. I started praying — all I could do was yell, 'Jesus!'" Allison said. "The doctor put his arm around my shoulder, 'Okay, mom, it's time for me to pull some strings. We're doing the surgery *now*.'"

Allison continued, "Suddenly, nurses shoved papers in my face to sign, and the bottom line, if I didn't choose surgery the outcome was death. I signed everything."

Immediately the word got out and the waiting room filled with family and friends — they hugged, some cried, and all prayed. As Allison and Jason stood in the circle of joined hands, the phone from the OR rang, "We're putting him on the heart/lung bypass," the most serious part of the surgery. Allison's sister started praying, "Please, Lord, increase his oxygen level and nourish his body." As the praying continued over the next two hours, the phone rang again. Allison picked up the phone and held it to her ear. "My sister's praying rang in one ear, and in the other ear I heard, 'His oxygen level is 94 percent, and he's off the heart/lung machine.' I'm sure people heard our shouts and 'amens' out on the street."

Over time, Nathan thrived, had another successful surgery, hit all the normal milestones, and turned three. Allison baked pies at Thanksgiving and took them to the nurse's station.

"Here's a small 'thank you' for the wonderful care we received here," she said. On their way out, Allison and Nathan stopped by the waiting room where other heart parents sat on those familiar couches, some leaned against the wall — curled up in blankets, Styrofoam cups of stale coffee littered the small tables — and others whispered to family and friends camped nearby.

"It's really hard sitting here, isn't it?" Allison said. The weary faces nodded. "We've been here, and let me introduce you to our son, Nathan." Nathan's bright brown eyes shone. He pulled up his shirt, "See my scar?" The weary parents indeed saw his scar, and *hope stood in front of them* — all three-and-a-half feet of that healthy boy with his huge smile.

What happened to the fairy tale? Fairy tales are make believe, but real life has easy times, and hard times (which often occur at the same time).

"That's just life here on earth," Allison said. The Wright's journey included Nathan's heart defect, two surgeries, three hospitalizations — and then Jason lost his job. When someone asked how he was doing while looking for another job, he answered, "God was with us every step with our son. I've trusted Him with our son; surely I can trust Him with something as minor as my job."

The heart journey winds through dark tunnels, and exits into sunlight — over and over again. All our journeys here on earth are guided by the engineer (God). Don't throw away your ticket and jump off. Sit still and trust that engineer.

Today, "Mr. Right" rides bikes with Caleb (HH), Nathan (HK), and Daniel (HH). And Allison pulls toddler Samuel (HH) in their red wagon. Here come the Wright brothers.

Single Caregivers: Alone in the Tunnel

"It's bad enough when you've heard those awful words while someone else is with you. But as a single parent sitting there all by yourself — I can't even describe it. You feel totally alone," a single caregiver said. The devastating diagnosis can leave single caregivers feeling besieged. How do they split their limited time? At work? With their child in the hospital? With the siblings at home? "There wasn't enough of me, and no one else to lean on. Money got tighter, I couldn't pay bills, and previous problems with my insecurities and fears shot to the surface."

As a single caregiver, you may feel as if everything lands on your shoulders. (You might flip over to Chapter Seven for helpful suggestions that deal with common problems of all caregivers.)

"I envy families who have support from other people. I'm in this by myself with my sick grandchild. Where do I go for help?"

As a single caregiver, you carry the weight of family decisions, but you need to share that load with others who come alongside. The following are suggestions from others who have walked this journey as a single caregiver — those who understand how you feel.

* Don't isolate yourself. Seek and join support groups for single caregivers at the hospital or online. They understand your difficult journey. Church groups and friends may not understand the difficulties, but they can provide emotional, physical, and spiritual help. Your time is limited and it's hard to carve out the hours for support, but make this a priority. Not only will this benefit you, but it will benefit your child as you are strengthened and encouraged.

Helps & Hope

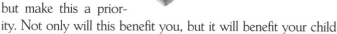

God's Word in the Tunnel

Dear caregivers, whatever your situation, hold on to this truth: God cares about you and your precious child. You can't be God for your children, but you can hand them over to Him. These are His words:
When you pass through the waters,
I will be with you;
And through the rivers, they shall not overflow you....
— Isaiah 43:2

He will be there.

* When your child was first admitted to the hospital, you probably received a notebook overflowing with information. If you can't find financial resource help, ask the hospital social worker to lead you to the assistance you need.

* Try to establish consistent daily routines. Even small amounts of time set aside can balance the stress of hospital, home, and work. A quick story before bedtime, a drive-thru meal together, or a telephone call at a specific time may bring security for you and your family — something to look forward to.

* Encourage consistent discipline of your child and their siblings by those who help you take care of them. Everyone needs to know how you want things done and it relieves second-guessing.

* Treat kids like kids, not a substitute for an adult partner. It's easy to put the oldest child into an adult role when you're exhausted and need help.

* Keep communication lines open with others through e-mails, CarePages, CaringBridge, and CareFlash sites (see Resource Three).

Reactions in the Tunnel

After the devastating diagnosis, most family members express these feelings:

* "Oh, God! I feel like I've been punched in the stomach."

* "I'm walking through a fog, sort of an out-of-body experience."

* "This can't be happening to my child." (shock).

But the real differences arise in the next steps as parents or caregivers seek to cope with an overwhelming situation. One mom said, "When we first heard the diagnosis, my husband, Tom, searched the Internet for days trying to find more information. I collapsed in tears trying to deny the diagnosis. How could we react so differently? He's *our* child."

The truth is that CHDs change the dynamics of the family. All members are still who they are, but their personalities become intensified. Weaknesses become more obvious, and strengths are often taken to the extreme in an attempt to cope. Unfortunately, even good things can be overdone. Some parents forage for information by searching the Internet. Some try to find help via chat rooms and sup-

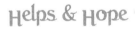

Helps & Hope

Others' reactions may not make sense to you, and honestly — in that moment — they may not make sense to the reactor either. But we're all entitled to feel what we feel.

port groups. Some shut down emotionally, and others cry or talk uncontrollably. Others' reactions may not make sense to you, but they make sense to the reactor. We all respond differently to stress.

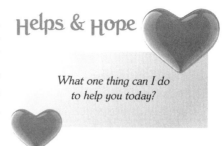

Helps & Hope

What one thing can I do to help you today?

In Tom's case his strength, searching for information, helped them make wise treatment decisions. His calm demeanor and task-oriented coping skills brought some control over the uncontrollable situation as they met with doctors. He compartmentalized his feelings and focused on his child's devastating diagnosis. However, Tom lost himself in the search for information and distanced himself from the family and his wife's emotions.

His wife, Janet, felt he pulled away and shut down when she needed him most. By contrast, she turned outward to others, communicating with hugs, tears, and talking to her network of friends and family. That network was already in place. Janet had reached out through her strengths to help others in need over the years. Now she needed much in return. Unfortunately, Tom was unable to express the emotions she needed from him, so she shut him out. Neither appreciated the strengths the other brought to the marriage, nor understood the other's behavior. Both ran on empty emotionally, with little to give the other as they dealt with the daily care of their sick child.

Sadly, the initial behavior, that starts out as a reaction to the shocking diagnosis, can harden into a pattern. Sometimes each spouse's coping mechanisms can result in the two parents pulling in opposite directions, whether consciously or subconscious to balance one another out. They may not realize that's what is happening — it just works that way many times. Take a few minutes to sit and talk face to face. Each asks, "What one thing can I do to help you today?" Then listen, without judgment, and try to do what was asked of you. These few minutes invested in each other will bring long-lasting rewards in filling those drained emotional tanks. There are exceptions to these rules. Some parents have expressed that rather than empty emotional tanks, their tanks felt overfilled with rage, fear, grief, and helplessness. To them, often, the idea of trying to communicate was overwhelming because opening that emotional valve might bring on more problems.

Also, see Resource One regarding "Love Languages" — how we give and receive love. Those suggestions may offer new insights for both of you.

You and your spouse have probably always had different parenting styles, but now those differences may seem magnified.

One frustrated dad said, "My wife smothers our daughter, so I have to balance it by being objective."

His wife's response? " 'Smothers?' She needs all my attention and I intend to give it to her."

Each partner pulled in the opposite direction trying to balance the situation and the result was an emotional tug-of-war. This is the kind of tension that builds up and hangs like invisible gas in the home. Then all it takes is the least spark — a harsh tone or rolling of the eyes — to ignite an explosion. Such a volatile atmosphere makes it nearly impossible to make the excruciating decisions that heart disease requires. The explosions can shake the entire family, and communication can further break down.

Take time to think about the coping mechanisms you are using. What about your spouse and the rest of your family? How is each person coping? Are empty emotional tanks creating a tug-of-war? Perhaps explosions aren't on your family's horizon, but you're both overwhelmed with sadness and have shut down so that you can deal with your own feelings. What can you do as a family to relieve some of the stress and strain of having a sick family member? Laughter helps. Can you find a funny movie to watch together? Or maybe even just watch silly clips on YouTube?

If your spouse or other family members are frustrating you, take time to consider that they, too, are just trying to cope with an overwhelming situation. They may not cope in the same way as you, but they're trying to make their way through. Ask God to show you their strengths, and then tell them you appreciate who they are and what they do. *It will be like cool water poured on parched ground.*

Talking in the Tunnel
Some parents are able to talk about their child and their feelings. The open dialogue brings them closer together. However, many

parents can't do this. They can discuss treatment plans with the doctors and carpool schedules with neighbors, but they fill every moment to avoid the main issue — their feelings about their child's diagnosis and treatment. They are treading water just to keep their heads above the surface — and that is a full-time job.

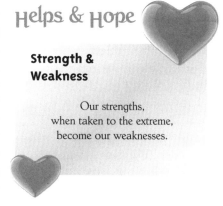

Helps & Hope

Strength & Weakness

Our strengths, when taken to the extreme, become our weaknesses.

One mom said, "Why didn't we talk about our child and our feelings? If we talked about it, it made it more real and the pain seemed twice as bad. So we didn't talk. And then we also ended up feeling abandoned by each other. We finally opened up, and what a relief to get those fearful feelings out. Since we had shared our fears once, we could do it again when needed."

That experienced mom had a few suggestions:

✳ Pray together each day about the situation. Ask God to lead your decisions and to give you strength. Express your fears openly to each other — as much as the other is comfortable in hearing it. (See Appendix One.)

✳ Express your fears openly to each other.

✳ Watch for opportunities to encourage each other when you're down.

Another mom said, "Talk and pray each day? I don't even have time to take a fast shower."

Sound familiar? When you think you have the least time for talking and praying is when you need it most. Don't let communication lapses continue. Every day that passes makes it more difficult to do. It may feel risky to reach out. You may find it easier to begin with a question. Ask your spouse about his or her fears, and *be sure to listen respectfully.* Don't judge and don't write off those fears as if they're not important.

As you think about bridging the communication gap, you may feel fearful that you'll be rebuffed by others who don't see the need for talking about the situation. It may seem easier to avoid the pain and hold your feelings inside, but it's worth taking the chance as walls come down and you connect emotionally with each other. However, be aware that some people can handle only a certain amount of information — Carepages, Caringbridge, and Careflash sites offer the outlet to give information and the "reader" can read and respond as they desire. Some want more details than others. They have different personalities and needs — uniquely made—just like you are.

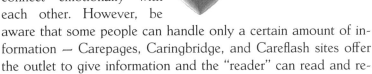

Helps & Hope

Speak Your Mind

There are no mind readers.
If you find yourself thinking,
he should know that I need...
No, he doesn't. Stop and tell him.
Let's look at some ways
we can get our emotional tanks
filled and how we can fill others'
tanks for the journey.

This journey is a marathon, not a dash, and daily decisions affect our relationships for the long haul. By choosing to encourage one another now — fill emotional tanks, and draw together, each step of the journey can at least be a little lighter. *Choose* to see whether you're discouraging your partner in some way, or draining your partner's emotional tank. If you don't make active *choices* to draw together, you may find yourselves drifting apart — even far apart.

Understanding Others in the Tunnel

Especially on this journey, communication is desperately needed with *all* the people in your life — family, friends, and hospital staff. Throughout this book, we refer to the You-niquely Made Personality Study, which highlights four basic personality types. (See Resource One for the whole study.) An understanding of personality types can help you enhance communication and fill others' empty emotional tanks. After a quick study of personality types, you may discover that your spouse, doctor, or sister isn't annoying you on purpose — it may simply be how they are "wired." This will help you identify strengths and weaknesses (your own and others') and provide some ideas about how to handle those weaknesses. Depending on personality type, different factors drain and fill emotional tanks. The heart journey is long and tanks need to be refilled — often. This study will help you do that.

The personality types in this study are color-coded because people connect emotionally to colors. Colors make it easier to remember the concepts — the outgoing Yellows, systematic Blues, driven Reds, and easygoing, shy, Greens.

One mom who read this study said, "That outgoing Yellow is so Kelly. That's why she's met everyone on the floor while I stayed in the room and hardly talked to our nurse. I feel more comfortable in mute-mode, I guess."

Most people say, "One of those colors is pretty much me, but I've also got a little of the others too."

Everyone is a unique combination of colors — a blend. Your emotional gene pool comes from both sides of your family. Some people think that males or females are only certain colors.

One husband said, "Women are so much more emotional than men. My wife overreacts to everything."

Of course, there are women and men in every color. A wife said, "My husband is the emotional one in our family. I'm the balanced one."

Some people seem to be one-color people, while others are combinations of several, but everyone needs acceptance for who they are, appreciation for what they do, and encouragement to keep on being and doing in their unique way.

Using Your You-niquely Made Personality Study

As you read the You-niquely Made Personality Study in Resource One, jot notes in the margins to jog your memory of who needs what. When you're exhausted, "color blindness" can cloud your perception. At those times it seems those optimistic Yellows aren't serious enough and don't follow through, the systematic Blues are too gloomy and nitpick every detail, the driven Reds don't care enough and boss others around, and the passive Greens don't show enough emotion and make napping an art form.

Look for the *positives* in each person to clear up that "color-blindness." A single positive comment can beam a ray of hope even in the darkest tunnel. And everyone can use all the rays they can get.

For I know the thoughts I think toward you,
says the LORD, the thoughts of peace and not of evil,
to give you a future and a hope.
Jeremiah 29:11

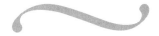

His half a heart has taught me to appreciate life with my whole heart.

— Heart mom

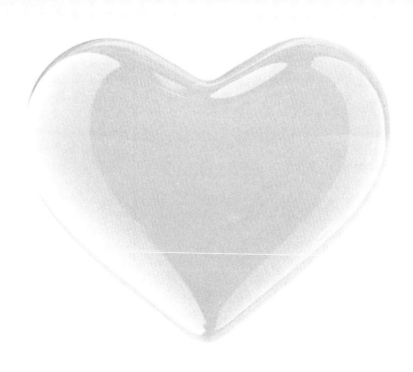

Chapter Three

What Do I Do Now?

Some Bonds Cannot Be Understood

Some bonds cannot be understood
Unless you have walked them before
A path that I would not have chosen
A future I just can't ignore.

We've all watched our children intently
Memorizing each line
And let them leave our loving arms
And prayed things would be fine.

We've paced the halls awaiting news
And wondered just what lies in store
We've felt our own heart's racing as
We walked through an ICU door.

We've seen the child we love so much
Struggling to overcome
The lines — the cords — the monitors
No thoughts — no words would come.

We've prayed for an improvement
We've laid it in God's hands
We've cried — we've hoped — we've worried
We've wondered about God's plans.

We've learned just how a heart works
Each valve and artery
We've asked a lot of questions
We've faced each surgery.

And somewhere down this well-worn path
We've met more families
Who know exactly what it means
To live with this disease.
We've smiled at every triumph
And shared in every sigh
We've prayed for a child that struggles
And each family that must say goodbye.

Some battles are fought with bullets
And weapons made for war
While these are fought in silence
Behind a hospital door.

We've wondered what lies in our future
We've been thankful for just one more day
We've stopped and watched with tear-filled eyes
Our children — as they play.

We've struggled with ounces and weight gain
Why won't my child just eat?
But heart moms — we're a tough group
We've learned how to face a defeat.

We've faced those moments others do
When life has got us stressed
But it doesn't take long to remember
That we are richly blessed.

We've taken on a whole new role
One we wouldn't exchange if we could
We know that life is difficult
We hold onto all that is good.

God chose each of us carefully
I do believe he smiled
Some bonds begin with strangers
And just one special child.

— Stephanie Husted, Heart mom

Through a Dad's Eyes

"I grew up on a 2,000 head cattle ranch in Oklahoma," Gregg said. "I just handled any problem that came along, because it was the cowboy's way of life. After I got married, I rode in rodeos for a living, then taught school and coached. I still thought I could handle anything. We had our first child, Jake, and a few years later our daughter, Jaycee. When she was a few months old, the control I *thought* I had over my life came to a screeching halt — she was diagnosed with a rare heart defect.

"Soon after the diagnosis, there my wife and I stood outside the operating room getting ready to give our tiny fragile daughter to the OR nurse."

Gregg looked down at that precious baby cradled in the palm of his calloused hand. The nurse smiled, and gently took Jaycee from him — then hit the entry button and went through the open steel doors.

"As those doors closed behind them — it hit. I wasn't in control of anything! That began my search for God. I figured He might have some control, and I needed Him."

Helps & Hope

We hand our children over to God — whether they are sick or well.

Through a Mom's Eyes

"It was time for my daughter Sarah's walk down the hall — which you'd think would've been simple. I climbed out of the recliner, unplugged the pumps from the outlets in the wall, maneuvered the IV poles and pumps — and shuffled down the hall. We made a loop around the nurse's desk — waved at them, then slowly walked back. When we got in the room, Sarah hoisted her exhausted body back into bed and I nestled into the chair. Just as she finally fell into a drugged sleep, the batteries beeped — I'd forgotten to plug all the pumps back in the wall outlets — and one was dying — loudly dying. So I climbed out of the recliner and searched behind the head of the bed for an empty outlet," Heather said.

"My mind was so tired I couldn't locate the empty one. I grabbed the headboard, jerked it with my right hand (still trying not to disturb Sarah), and then wedged my left hand to search down the wall. The more I searched, the more the tears came to the surface, and I finally just plopped down on the floor. Through my tears, there it was — the illusive outlet down near the bottom of the wall. I stuck the plug into the socket and breathed a deep sigh — then pulled myself up and collapsed in the recliner (thankful I *had* a chair that reclined), when I heard a whisper."

"Mommy, I need to go to the bathroom." Heather leaned forward in her chair and attempted to untangle the spaghetti of IV lines. "Never mind," Sarah said. "I don't have to go now," and she buried her face in her fuzzy heart bear.

Heather continued, "Actually, that was one of the easier things we accomplished that evening, and I don't know why that outlet was so major — well, I do know. When you're exhausted, frustrated, and worried about your child, even the small things

Helps & Hope

Save Your Energy

Keep your eye on the gas gauge. Fill up when you're approaching a quarter of a tank. Don't push it to the "E." You never know when you'll need to make a trip to the ER, especially in the middle of the night.

seem huge at the time." Heather fell asleep — at least until the next beep.

What do you do *for* that uniquely made child? The following chapter gives help for different ages, stages, and situations in which you deal with your precious child.

But seek first the kingdom of God and His righteousness, and all these things shall be added unto you.
Matthew 6:33

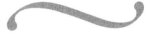

When you pass through the waters, I will be with you;
And through the rivers, they shall not overflow you....

— Isaiah 43:2

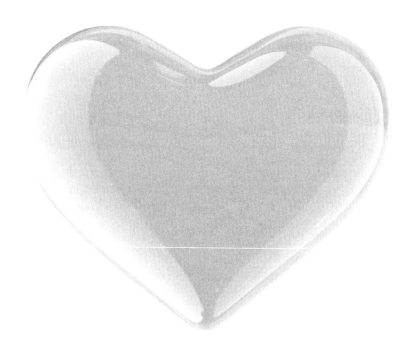

Chapter Four

Caring For Your Unique Child

What do thumbprints, snowflakes, and children have in common? They're unique — no two thumbprints, snow-flakes, or children are exactly the same. You can't be "sort of" unique says the dictionary. Unique is absolute, and your child is absolutely him or herself — with a mixture of age, personality, and now diagnosis. Let's begin with the ages and stages your child goes through in their one-of-a-kind way.

Ages and Stages

We all know that children progress through stages as they mature. That doesn't change just because a child has a heart defect. HKs go through these stages with the added variables of surgeries, treatments, and short- and long-term side effects. Whether your HK is a baby, teen, somewhere in-between, or an adult "child," you may want to read each of the age-group sections. Your family has expanded on this journey and now includes other parents and their HKs. Any advice you can share

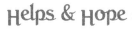

Helps & Hope

They mainly want you to be there for them.

with other families regarding their children will be valuable — as all of you deal with many new normals.

"What are the typical issues that children go through at different ages?" I asked several heart moms and medical professionals. The same answer kept popping up, "One size does not fit all. There are so many variables, but generally, if you get through the preschool years, then your child's elementary years go fairly well. You may have other issues later, but each child — their diagnosis — their personality — their family life, all are things which impact each year of life." Remember as you read this next section that **one size doesn't fit all**.

Of course, the best advice is what you already know. All children — whatever their age, whether sick or well — need love. They mainly want you to be there for them.

Infants and Toddlers

This age learns through their five senses, and they live in the now. "Ones" toddle (anywhere they can). "Twos" trample (anything in sight). As the toddler adds a hearty, "No!" he wields power over those big people who chase him, pull objects out of his mouth, and grab him as he heads for the stairs or street.

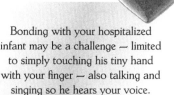

Helps & Hope

Bonding with your hospitalized infant may be a challenge — limited to simply touching his tiny hand with your finger — also talking and singing so he hears your voice. Ask the nurse for suggestions.

Each child has his own individual timetable when he will do things. However, two important characteristics develop during these years: curiosity and exploration. It's that running, climbing, and stuffing-everything-in-the-mouth phase. Despite your exhaustion from corralling your toddler, take advantage of the times with your HK is in the hospital, clinic, or at home. Rock her (if she'll hold still), read to her, look into her eyes, talk and sing to her. Children this age love music, and they think Mom or Dad's singing voice is great — no matter what.

Helps & Hope

The best and most beautiful things in the world cannot be seen or even touched. They must be felt with the heart.
Helen Keller

"Kaiser was the biggest baby in the nursery, over eight pounds, and chubby-cheeked, we never suspected a thing would be wrong," his mom said. "Later when he was lying next to the other heart babies, he looked huge. Most were so tiny and fragile, some struggling for life."

"Heart infants' first year of life is difficult because they can get tired easily, especially while trying to nurse or take a bottle. It took my precious baby girl over two hours to take two ounces of milk," a mom said. "Bless her heart, she was so fussy, but if we let her cry she turned blue."

"Heart toddlers *do* stuff everything in their mouths," a heart mom said. Some do have food aversions, but some not — just like other toddlers! And these babies still learn like other babies — with their senses. And learn with a lot of love.

Three- to Six-year-olds

Three- to six-year-old children are concrete thinkers and link illness with specific actions. They believe if they do certain things, then certain things will follow. For instance, if you take medicines, you feel better. When other children this age learn of your child's heart defect, they may think they can "catch" it. And, your child may think she can give it to others. The concept that a heart defect can't be "caught" needs to be explained by parents, teachers, coaches, and anyone who interacts with your child and other children around your child.

Children this age feel that the world revolves around them and they are in control of what happens. Just because they may use some of the big words (the heart jargon they pick up), it doesn't mean they know what it is and what it does. They need a lot of age-appropriate information and reassurance from adults. It is difficult to explain things to these concrete-thinkers, but remember to turn to the hospital's child life specialist if you have questions or concerns.

One mom said, "My five-year-old spouts off the names of her meds to any medical student who comes in the room."

This is her new world and her new words. The main thing children this age want is love and attention from their parents. They can get upset when ignored, so remember how important it is to work and play with your child at this age. They *like* to help adults, so give them opportunities to fold clothes, bring you something from another room, or help pack a lunch. Being needed and appreciated can help fill emotional spaces treatments may have sapped.

Even young children can feel depressed if left out of activities with friends. A weak immune system, hospitalizations, and fatigue can take their toll on friendships. It will be up to you to create opportunities for him or her to interact with other children. Invite one friend at a time to play outside, (indoor activities may breed bacteria), and ask your child what she'd like to do — which may bring a smile to her face and lift her spirits.

Even at this age, you can start talking to your child about his or her heart defect, but try to keep it matter of fact as you discuss meds, doctor's appointments and other issues woven into his daily life.

Seven- to Eleven-year-olds

The world of a child in this age group is ever expanding to friends, teachers, and coaches who are important to them. Keep these people in the loop through calls and e-mails. People want to help. Let them know the best way to reach out to your child.

The HK wants to be "normal" and fit in with a group. Being different in any way — how she looks, aptitude in class, the ability to participate in playground games, or missing school — may bring on teasing or unwanted attention. Be on the lookout for that, and ask others (teachers in particular) to do the same.

This is probably a fairly smooth time in your child's life, once again depending on his diagnosis. Of course, your doctor's recommendations as to his exercise will be helpful for you as the parent — the parent who has been guiding, protecting, and watching over your child. It may be difficult to "let go" in many ways during these years, but the "letting go" is part of the journey. One cardiology chaplain said, "These kids need to learn to live in the real world. Momma isn't always going to be there, and it may be hard for momma to let go because she's been needed and has been her child's biggest advocate through a horrendous journey."

One HK (who was more restricted) said, "At least I could be involved in *Jump Rope for Heart*, even though I couldn't jump. My friends really liked being able to help me that way — to raise money — and I could tell them more about what it was like to have a heart defect."

As a parent, you know at this age his friends are extremely important to him, but you still count too. He may be worried that he won't fit in with his friends, afraid that they'll forget him, and not sit with him at lunch when he goes back to school if he's had to be out for a while. It's been a long time since you were eight, but you remember those concerns. Anything that sets you apart from your peers can be a real negative — even something you have no control over, like a chronic illness or its side effects. Keep the communication lines open with your uniquely made child.

You are your child's advocate.

If needed, one Special Education Advocate advises parents to explore Physical Education and other modifications for their child at school under "Other Health Impaired" through the federal IDEA (Special Education) guidelines. You will have to check your state's Department of Public Instruction laws regarding what modifications can be made for your child — and don't take the first "no" as the answer. Federal Title 504 also is available to offer modifications, as well, in many cases.

Ask your doctor what kinds of activities are appropriate for your child. If modifications are called for, ask him or her to write a prescription spelling out your child's needs, then contact your school district office and speak to the Director of Pupil Services/Special Education Director to make the referral.

Teens

Changes occur rapidly during the middle school years (ages twelve to fourteen). Hormones kick in, which affect their bodies *and* their emotions. Teens in good health experience a kaleidoscope of emotions and opinions that can vary from day to day. A teen grappling with a life-threatening illness may experience that kaleidoscope more intensely. Many teens this age are quite empathetic; teens on a heart journey may become even more so. Those friends who look past your HK's "differences" may become steadfast friends, so help your HK keep those friends in the loop with day-to-day happenings.

Helps & Hope

Don't throw away your friendship with your teenager over behavior that has no great moral significance. There will be plenty of real issues that require you to stand like a rock. Save your big guns for those crucial confrontations.
— Dr. James C. Dobson

Be aware that it's not uncommon for some friends to back away from your HK (not knowing how to handle the situation). If that happens, your HK may withdraw. Keep your eyes open to the social impact of your HK's health situation and don't shy away from discussing it.

Like most teens, HKs don't want to be different from their friends. Look at how most teens dress and talk — just like their friends. Now add some med's side effects to those everyday teen pressures and consider what your teen may be grappling with. If your teen is asking to stay home from school, try to glimpse the story behind the story. What's going on? Encourage school attendance as much as possible in order to keep up with work and stay connected with friends. Each middle school situation is unique, and may be difficult to adjust to at best, *without* the added stresses of heart defects. Ask for help when needed with counselors and child life specialists. Your teen may need to talk through the various reactions they get from friends — positive and negative. And that's okay.

Whatever the age of your teen, encourage him or her to reach out to younger HKs who respond to the "big kids."

"Sometimes they relate to them better than the adult professional staff," a nurse said and smiled.

This interaction gets teens outside themselves. The truth is that everyone needs to be needed.

Helps & Hope

Encourage your teen (as young as thirteen) to begin taking responsibility for her health care — gradually preparing her for adulthood.

As teens transition to high school (ages fifteen to eighteen), their world may become more social, and they will begin to experience greater concerns about driving and dating. Those concerns may seem frivolous to adults when there's a CHD diagnosis in the picture, but that's the world of teens. Friends can do a lot to infuse strength.

Your teen is two people in one. One needs independence to fly, and the other needs the security of a nest in which to rest. Those conflicting needs can cause a lot of confusion for teens and their families.

Teens know what they're missing in life, and depression can quickly set in. Hospital staff members and other teens can cut through walls teens may build, perhaps more easily than parents can. Support groups for these "almost" adults are valuable. Support groups are valuable for their parents too. This journey is difficult for both. Teens think in terms of symptoms and side effects — how they affect their everyday lives and their futures. They realize the importance of the treatments, even if they don't like them.

Helps & Hope

Teens need to be reminded about the importance of their choices.

However, at times teens need to be reminded about the importance of their choices.

Sometimes they will be tempted to go to an activity and not tell anyone (especially their mom) how sick they are. Having "head knowledge" (logic) doesn't necessarily override "heart's desire," (emotion). That kind of wisdom only comes with maturity. To them, a fever isn't worth missing a game, party, or some other fun event.

Helps & Hope

Alert!

Be sure your HK takes dental hygiene seriously — check with your cardiologist to find out if antibiotics are needed before dental procedures.

Have conversations with your teen about the results of body piercings, drinking, smoking, and sex. Results are *especially* serious for an HK. You may need to enlist someone else from your child's life or a trusted nurse to get through to him the importance of the *long run*. Even teens with heart defects can feel indestructible; they need information from a trusted source so they can understand how a spiked fever — as well as choices they make — can drastically affect that long run.

Young Adults

There's a *new*, new normal for 500,000 young adults in the United States. With improved surgical and medical care of children with CHD over the past 50 years, an ever-increasing number of patients have reached adult life and require informed long-term medical follow-up and supportive services.

"They should be considered a new cardiovascular sub-specialty — but aren't most of the time — because with an acute medical crisis and after cardiac surgery, they may be hospitalized on a pediatric unit, an adult unit, or *both* during a hospital(s) stay," experts say.

Teens and young adults with CHD grapple with the same issues of identity as their non-CHD counterparts: positive body image, envisioning adult roles and responsibilities, expanding peer relationships, sexual intimacy/fertility, establishing a value system based on their own beliefs, and trying to move toward more autonomous control over their lives. Their lives with CHD has been all they've known — and they have acquired knowledge of their disease, meds, and what may happen — as well as awareness of the uncertainty of the future. A "You're doing well," statement from their doctor may be heard as

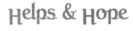

Helps & Hope

By the way, your child is your child, no matter what age, said a heart mom, about her fifty-year-old **child**.

"Not good enough" to the patient. Everything is relative, and they may need more input and counseling to deal with all the unasked-for variables in their lives.

During a hospital stay in a pediatric unit which is set up for babies and children — young adults' size, age, and wanting to have a say in their care may be difficult for the nursing staff.

"Younger children take the meds given, and adjust to what needs to be done, because we are the adults and we say so. We've worked with these babies and children for so long — we just know what to do, most of the time," a pediatric cardiac nurse said. "We try to get the adult patient out to the adult unit or home as soon as possible for their sake."

When the young adult is moved to an adult unit, or even starts out there, what are the challenges? "No one seemed to know what to do with me," a patient said. "They kept thinking I was asking for too much pain medication, but I know what's worked in the past. They were used to older heart patients with different problems, and CHD's weren't seen that often."

"We have so much to do with our regular patients, that it's like learning a new disease, meds, and also, we're not used to the parents being vocal in their *child's* care — and the *child* being so knowledgeable either," a cardiac nurse said.

Next steps come: how do you as a parent handle your child's moving away?

"People asked how we could let our daughter go away to college? I answered, 'How could we *not* let her go?' It's hard to have them away from you if something were to happen, but life can't stop — especially if they have desires to pursue their dreams — even if it's away from you," a heart mom said. "She's dealt with this disease and has had input in her care for years now."

Vocations for CHD's? For most people with congenital heart defects, job choices aren't limited. Young adults with heart defects have entered a variety of professions and occupa-

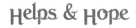

Helps & Hope

Children in a family are like flowers in a bouquet: there's always one determined to face in an opposite direction from the way the arranger desires.
— Marcelene Cox

tions as high school and college counselors help a person select a vocation. Sometimes the state vocational rehabilitation program may be needed for those rare patients whose ability to earn an income has been impaired by a physical handicap due to a heart problem.

Personality

Each age and stage brings so many changes; however, your child is always uniquely him or herself — a blend of colors from that personality gene pool.

As we've discussed, understanding personality types can help make this journey a little easier. Keep the types in mind as you deal with your HK and encounter others along the way. (Don't forget to turn to Resource One for more information.)

Some are wired to do the opposite of whatever you want, others can't wait to please you, and some seem to be in another world — but all are uniquely made — and need love.

Yellows

Yellows not only see the glass half full — but overflowing. They want people around 24/7. They're emotional, but they're also resilient. They may be crying one minute, but they bounce back quickly — especially if there are people involved. Adding steroids to these high-energy children? Tighten your grip as the roller coaster dives and jerks, but know that this too shall pass when the steroids are finished.

Encourage your Yellow's smile and outgoing personality and help them understand what a gift that is to others, especially in hospitals. Yellows can brighten everyone else's day, making twenty best friends on the first lap around the nurse's station. Again, Yellows need to receive hugs, positive comments, and attention — and they will give the same to others.

Blues

Blues tend to see the glass half empty. They feel pain more deeply and expect the worst will happen. "That last test hurt, so this one will for sure." They like things done in order, so make charts that show progress. Depending on your child's age, use smiley faces or other positive reinforcements after treatments, tests, and doctor and hospital visits. Let your child choose the stickers, realizing of course the length of time it will take in picking out the *perfect* ones. Thank Blues for the ways they take care of things. "His room looks like my office, but more organized," one doctor whispered about his Blue patient. Having an organized room will fill any Blue's emotional tank. They need to hear they've made a positive difference in other's lives. "Tyler down the hall, really appreciated the game you shared with him," a mom said. They also need to experience getting out of themselves and giving to others. Encourage that throughout their lives, and especially now.

Reds

Reds couldn't care less if there's a glass, but if there is, they want to be in control of it. They direct others — the hospital staff included.

"My daughter's been waited on hand and foot in the hospital and assumes that should continue at home. We had a battle royal getting her to pick up toys in her room. Fortunately, I'm as strong-willed as she," a Red mom said. "The good part is these strong-willed children persevere when others give up, and that's a plus in this world of heart disease."

If a parent is an exhausted, low-energy Blue or Green, she may give in regarding rules with medication and other procedures.

"Everything seems like a major deal," a weary parent said. Hang in there and choose your battles. Let the Red child have input and control when that's possible. They need that feeling. However, the battles you choose to win will give your strong-willed Red child boundaries and security.

Greens

Rather than experiencing the glass as half empty or as half full, Greens say, "What glass?"

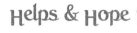

Helps & Hope

Our main business is not to see what lies dimly at a distance but to do what lies clearly at hand.
— Thomas Carlyle

Greens are sometimes overlooked because they don't demand attention as do the Reds and Yellows. If the parent is a self-starting Yellow or Red, a Green child simply follows their lead and instruction. Because they're content to be inactive, Greens need to be prompted to get physical (to whatever extent is approved by the medical staff) and mental exercise. Hours spent watching TV or sleeping can be counterproductive in the treatment program. Also, because Greens are accustomed to others making decisions for them, they need to be encouraged to take ownership in the treatment regimen. If you have a Green, discuss options with her and let her make those decisions (as are age-appropriate).

Of course, if you're a Red parent, you'll find it difficult to abide by those decisions. However, the results will be good for her *and* good for you. She needs to take more control over her life, and you need to give it to her.

Helping Your Unique Child

We've talked about your unique child's age and personality. Now here are some more tools to add to your caregiver's toolbox in helping your HK.

Emotional Help

Whether you are currently in a new place, with new people and procedures for your HK, or you're the seasoned veterans, all children need stress relievers. Help them get the endorphins flowing to tell their brain they feel better. Read the section on endorphins in Chapter Seven. Teach your child deep breathing techniques, squeezing a small ball to reduce stress, closing their eyes and imagining where they'd like to be, exercising (even wiggling toes and lifting their arms is a start), listening to favorite music, and laughing. Child life specialists are great resources for helpful hints and ideas.

Providing a feeling of control over the situation can also help your child's emotional health. Depending on your child's age, your child should be part of the team that discusses their type of heart defect, treatment, medicines, and side effects. You can also talk with your child about the timing of tests and treatments. In an uncontrollable situation, even a calendar can help. You might say, "You pick out the calendar that you want to use so we can mark the days of doctor's visits, treatment, or tests." Most children feel as if they have some control while marking off the days. However, don't tell younger children too far in advance about upcoming treatments, it may make them anxious because they have little understanding of time. How far in advance depends on the age and personality of your child. Make the calendar milestones a positive event for those sensitive Blues who've made an art form of worrying. Again, you know your child the best, and what will work for him or her.

Another way to give your child a feeling of control over his or her treatment is to allow the child to answer the doctor's questions directly, *before* you jump in with the "right" answer. This is not always easy to do. You understand better what the doctor was asking about the technical aspects of your HK's condition, but allowing them to answer first is very empowering, and helps them to know their feelings matter to you — that you respect how they feel and what they're thinking. Even a very young child can say, "I feel good!" or, "I feel tired."

Discipline

Rules convey a sense of normalcy. By sticking to your family's rules, you will be helping your child. Of course, as we've seen, some children more easily comply with rules than others. Some, such as strong-willed Red children, are naturally more challenging — and can find ways to push the limits — even between bouts of throwing up!

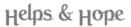

Helps & Hope

Discourage your child from running up and down the halls an hour after having chest tubes removed — and good luck with that! Someone said, "Firmness shows respect for you, friendly shows respect for them."

After a heart diagnosis, some parents wonder whether they should discipline their child, at all. Some people say you can't spoil a heart kid, and others say you can. Child life therapists tell parents, "If it was wrong before a heart diagnosis, it's wrong during one."

They have seen the effects of spoiling — when the child becomes self absorbed, the parents feel guilt for never doing enough (emotional blackmail by HK), and siblings who crave attention and seldom get their fair share. Let's face it. Disciplining healthy children can be a challenge. Parents who have children with a chronic illness have a lot of reasons why they don't discipline or set limits. Here are a few:

* "It's hard to say no when your child has thrown up for hours."

* "When you're exhausted, it's just easier to give in."

* "I don't know which behaviors are related to his heart and which aren't."

All these are valid reasons, especially when you're physically and emotionally drained.

Take an attitude check — the *child's* attitude. Does he control decisions that you should be making? Is your child reacting one way in the hospital and another heading toward a favorite fast food place?

Some parents say, "If I discipline my child I'm afraid he won't love me as much."

This isn't about your child filling *your* needs. This concerns your *child* needing boundaries (rules) that only you can give. Rules create security and a sense of normalcy, whether he realizes it or not. When the rules remain the same even though the situation has changed, you are sending the message that life goes on, and we do, too. That's our new normal. We are still a family and families still have rules. Consistency creates security.

Do you think the demanding child, usually a controlling Red, whose room has more toys than the hospital gift shop will curb expectations when you go home? If a child can get anything she wants in the hospital, why not continue to demand the same at home, school, with grandparents, whomever they're with, and wherever they are?

"No one wants to be around a spoiled child — heart kid or not," a parent said.

That's especially true for the child's siblings who often feel left out.

"I wish I was the sick one so I get new toys," a sibling said.

When you're a six-year-old sibling, you only see the "good" things the sick child gets.

So what happens next? Some parents try to give the siblings equal gifts to even things out. If you have several other children, it really adds up.

"Where does this stop?" a mom asked.

"I guess it stops when we say so," the dad responded under his breath.

Whether your child has siblings or he's an only child, gifts are appropriate — occasionally — just make sure they aren't overdone.

A friend told the following story:

One day I was talking to another mom who was mentoring me with my chronically ill daughter. The other mom laughed when I told her I was torn about discipline. "Oh, listen, I've been down that road. When our third son was two, he just wasn't growing like he should have been — wasn't thriving. We took him to the doctor, and long story short, he only had one functioning kidney — and it wasn't functioning well. We were devastated. I made up my mind that, for as long as God allowed us to have him, he was going to be happy. Whatever he wanted he was going to get. If he wanted ice cream three

Spoiling Them

It is not giving children more that spoils them; it is giving them more to avoid confrontation.
— John Gray

meals a day then that was fine with me. And I was never going to tell him 'no' again. Well, it didn't take long before his brothers despised him, and resented us for over-indulging him and for letting him get away with murder. After a particularly difficult day with the boys, my husband and I looked at each other and said, 'that child is running us like a couple of trick ponies.' I wanted him to be a happy, but he wasn't happy being in charge. The normal order of things had been turned upside-down when we abdicated power to him. Our sunny little boy had turned into a sullen dictator, and we had allowed it to happen. The next day, we went about changing things back to our old routine. He kicked and screamed and carried on like any (by that time) three-year-old does when they don't get their way, but, with consistency, we got our sunny little boy back, and our family got on with being 'normal' again."

Need help with appropriate discipline, and how much gift-giving to do? Talk to your child life specialist and other professionals. They've seen it all and are valuable resources.

Spiritual Help

People were bringing little children to Jesus to have him touch them, but the disciples rebuked them. When Jesus saw this, he was indignant. He said to them, "Let the little children come to me, and do not hinder them, for the kingdom of God belongs to such as these. I tell you the truth, anyone who will not receive the kingdom of God like a little child will never enter it."

And he took the children in his arms, put his hands on them and blessed them.
~ Mark 10:13-16

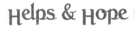

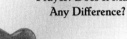
Because of this demanding journey, parents may only focus on the physical and emotional parts of the child. Don't neglect the part you can't see — the spiritual.

Praying (simply talking to God) with your child each day connects your child with Him. Your child learns to walk, talk, and become a person by mimicking you. Keep in mind that much is caught, not taught. They grow in their spiritual life much the same way. Your life is the lesson they're learning.

Your unique child may live in a new room — a hospital room — for a while. The following chapter gives hints from those who've made those new rooms home. Even small items brought from home make a huge difference — home to "home."

✳

Finally,...be strong in the Lord and in the power of His might.
Ephesians 6:10

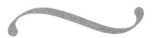

Through the LORD's mercies we are not consumed,
Because His compassions fail not. They are new every morning;
Great is Your faithfulness.

— Lamentations 3:22-23

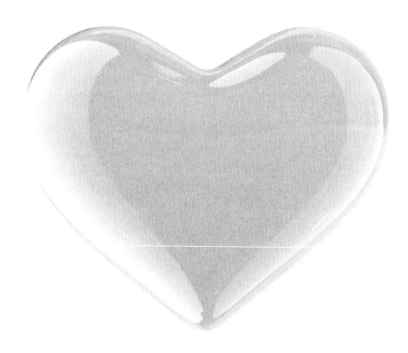

Chapter Five

Making Your Hospital Room Home

"We've earned frequent flyer status at our child's hospital."

You're heading to the hospital (again) so have a well-stocked "carry on" to grab as you go out the door. What necessities have you packed? You'll need things for yourself, your child, and depending on the age of your child — things to make the room "home" in different ways.

It's not easy to feel comfortable in the hospital, but it will be a bit easier if you make your child's hospital room feel homey.

One mom said, as she and her child left the hospital, "I won't miss those four white walls."

If you're living with four white walls or fortunate enough to have a color-decorated children's hospital room, making it home helps your stay. Mostly it helps everyone's mental health. Before you set about the task, make sure you ask about the hospital's rules.

Frequency?

Some heart defects require brief, infrequent hospital stays, but some require longer and more frequent stays. This chapter gives helpful hints for both journeys.

First Things First

First things first. Bring your HK's favorite blankets (quilts), pillow, and stuffed animals from home. The key word is *favorite*. Age doesn't seem to make a difference here. Teens need security blankets also (and so do adults). When you're nestled in the hospital bed, it's comforting to finger the softness of your familiar blanket and snuggle your face into your pillow that smells like home.

"What is something special you've had over your twenty-four years with a CHD?" I asked Jaycee.

"You won't believe this, but I still carry a special blanket (now a shred of material) and a baby doll (that looks worse for the wear) every time I go to the hospital. I've had ten surgeries, twenty procedures, and months, off and on, in various hospitals since I was three-and-a-half weeks old. Dorothy, the dear lady who made that blanket years ago, keeps saying, 'I'll make you a new one,' but this one is my comfort — and the doll."

Decorating Hints

Here are a few ways that your decorations can assist the staff and visitors.

Place a sign on the door to let others know how your child feels that day. Have your child draw simple faces with a smile or frown and place an arrow with a fastener in the middle, then you can point the arrow to the "feeling" of the hour. You can also add any special messages as this is a great tool for facilitating communication. You might also consider placing your child's name in large letters above the head of the bed, like this: Hi! My name is Julie! The sign will help everyone coming in the room, and it's nice for your child also.

Decorating the walls (if it's allowed) — Butterflies? Batman? Boats? What's your child's favorite? Let him decide the theme and give him suggestions on how it can be done (as much as is permitted). Also, if you're in and out of the hospital a lot, change the themes. Have your child choose as many of the things displayed as possible. Themes don't have to be costly. Display your child's art creations, coloring-book pictures of the theme, balloons, and toys from home.

Helps & Hope

Cheer Up!

Your homey hospital room can cheer up the patient, family, friends, and staff. Everyone can use some cheering up.

Also, siblings can color pictures and help with decorations. If you're putting pictures on the walls, avoid cellophane tape, which can pull off paint. Use poster tack instead, or whatever the hospital suggests.

Time can lose all meaning in the hospital so put up a schedule for the day. If your child feels well enough, have her check off (or use stickers to mark) what's been done during the day. This gives her a feeling of accomplishment. The schedule tells your child what to do and when to do it during the day and evening. Your child may find it easier to obey the schedule that tells her what to do rather than obey you. And you'll get a break from repeating, "It's time to...."

After a few days (which may seem like weeks or months), both of you will have every detail of the room memorized. A change will help — however slight that may be. Moving chairs, tables, signs on the walls, will be simple. However, if you want to move the bed for more open floor space, ask permission to do so. It may or may not be possible to do that.

Give the scary IV pole and pump a nickname, then decorate it. Tie balloons on it; drape it with colored streamers; hang stuffed animals on it. Camouflage is the key. Others will enjoy seeing the decorated pole and pump maneuvered

Helps & Hope

Give the scary IV pole and pump a nickname, then decorate it.

down the hall by your HK or as it simply decorates the room.

Balloons sent by friends or family are special and they make wonderful decorations. Tie them to the bed or the IV pole; you can also attach them to walls. Remember; choose Mylar balloons, not Latex. (Some people are allergic to Latex.) Cards also make wonderful decorations. Hang them on your walls or stick them between the blinds on the window. Save them for later to put in a scrapbook. Photos make some of the best decorations. **Display pictures of your family — including your pets.** Put up pictures that show your HK when he or she was healthy. It's great for others to see, and it's wonderful for you to remember and look forward to again. If you think your child is in need of a laugh, ask friends and family to take some pictures making funny faces. When your child is napping, put the funny photos up as a surprise.

Consider hanging a huge blank piece of paper or poster board for people to sign their names and write messages to your HK. Encourage staff to sign it too. Title it, "My Visitors." Your HK will love the positive messages written especially for them.

Similarly, for older children and teens, purchase an inexpensive journal and have visitors and staff "sign in" and write a personal message there. These make wonderful keepsakes and can follow your child from hospital stay to hospital stay, depending on the size of the journal.

Hints for Passing the Time

Time can move slowly in the hospital, and it may take a little creativity to find enjoyable ways to spend time together — and apart. Here are a few ideas.

✳ Enjoy a picnic — on the bed, floor, or tray table — just so you're with the one you love. Be thankful for the food you have, and on special nights order in pizza. "Even Jell-O shared together can be special," a mom said.

✳ Puzzles and games help keep minds sharp and encourage interaction with others. Bring your favorite games from home, or borrow some from the child life specialist.

✳ Need a diversion? Watch TV or movies.

* Listen to CDs and iPods. Have headphones handy and put them on for others who need silence — especially if the other person needs a nap.

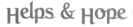
Helps & Hope

God invites us to take a holiday (vacation), to stop being God for a while and let him be God.
— Simon Tugwell

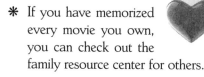

* If you have memorized every movie you own, you can check out the family resource center for others.

* Take photos or bring some from home and start a scrapbook. Or you could take photos and make a collage of pictures of staff and other HKs and their families as they come and go.

* Touch the world with the Internet. Many hospitals have e-mail connections. Computers equipped with Web cams, microphones and speakers can help children have real time interaction from their hospital room or their home with friends, relatives and classmates. Web cams with microphones can be purchased from local computer or office supply stores. There are several online services that offer the ability to video conference with your loved ones. SKYPE (www.skype.com) is free software that works seamlessly with your Internet connection. You can chat away with free Skype-to-Skype calls and never worry about cost, time nor distance.

* Also, handheld computerized games can be used most anywhere.

* Tack favorite Bible verses and sayings on a poster board to see first thing in the morning and whenever your child (or you) need a reminder of His love.

Make some art. Cut up old calendars with special pictures and make collages. After getting permission, paint windows with washable markers made for glass. Art is a great way to get out feelings. It's good for your child and for the family. You could even try pounding Play-Doh™ or clay for an emotional release. Want a blessing? Make something for somebody else.

Bring your favorite books from home. Check in the family resource center, which probably has shelves of books you've never seen.

Don't forget to create a quiet space. Sometimes a child needs to be alone. Set aside a corner of the room for this. Turn down the lights and add soft music.

Celebrate special occasions or holidays with strings of garland around the room. Choose colors that go with that holiday or your child's favorite colors. Just celebrate. Display your cards on a clothesline tied across the room. If it is Christmas, decorate a small tree. A ceramic tree will do. Here's another suggestion, decorate your IV pole and pump as a tree.

Give parties for milestones accomplished. Even small steps are steps. Celebrate with family, friends, and staff.

Tips for the Caregiver

When you're the caregiver and you're watching your child cope with such a challenge, it's easy to forget yourself. But living at the hospital is tough on you too. Here are some suggestions from caregivers who've lived in the new home. Don't forget to bring the following items from home in your "carry on."

If you're a new mommy you may need these extra items:

✳ Breast pump

✳ Pads

✳ Pillow to sit on

✳ Extra vitamins

✳ Support hose (if needed) to keep legs from swelling

✳ And, at times, hugs from anyone passing by.

New mommy, your hormones are in a state of flux which affects your body and emotions. Give yourself time to adjust, and if the tears flow "for no reason" you have added "reason" with a heart baby. Post partum is a change, and post partum with a heart baby is even more so.

Now for the regular items:

* Toiletries (necessities!)

* Your meds. "Since my child's heart defect was the biggie, I ignored my pains — like a toothache, PMS, and meds I was on. But that catches up after a while," a mom said.

* Jot notes on things happening to you and what you can do about them.

* Wear warm socks or house shoes, comfortable clothes, and bring a sweater or jacket — rooms sometimes are very cool — and you are sitting for long periods of time.

* Pictures of family (be sure they have pictures of you and your HK at home)

* Camera (ready for candid shots)

* Water bottles (you can refill them at the sink)

* A special mug for teas and coffee (keep tea bags, hot chocolate, and coffee handy) — plastic, insulated mugs keep hot drinks hot and cold drinks cold.

* Healthy snacks (to balance out all the others)

* Magazines, books, videos, DVDs, CDs and CD player (with earphones) or an MP3 player . With the whooshing of oxygen and beeping of monitors, your eyes and ears are bombarded with noise and blinking lights. "Is that sound good or

bad news? Is my baby in distress?" Ask a nurse, then put on some soothing, uplifting music — *good noise.*

* Journal (for the journey)

* Glasses (and an extra pair if you have one)

* Pillow and a quilt (you need a "blankie" too)

* Thank you notes to slip to others while you're in your new "home" (pray to see their needs through God's eyes)

* Your own unique things to make the room feel homier for you

* List of names, phone numbers, and e-mails addresses to keep in touch with everyone

* List of who is doing what and who you need to thank for helping your family

* Calendars, pencils, pens, and stickers (you could use some smiley-face stickers too)

* Your Bible and a devotional book (a suggested list of these books is in Resource Two)

* Put Bible verses and quotes on cards to set out or stick on the mirror (you never know when you might need the encouragement).

Having everything you need on hand in the hospital room will make you more comfortable and help you to feel some control. Keep your calendar/journal and pen handy as you schedule things and keep track of your family at home. Contact information for family and friends is invaluable. It's easy to forget even familiar phone numbers when you're stressed and running on empty.

Friends can't surround you physically at all times, but try to stay in touch through phone calls, e-mails, and notes. Put up notes received, especially if your child is in isolation.

Here are a few more suggestions for you, the caregiver, to help life run as smoothly as possible during a bumpy time.

Helps & Hope

Tips 'n Tricks

Find "homes" for the many new papers and items on this new journey.

* Leave recipes and helpful hints for Mr. Mom at home — or whoever is there. Keep a list of any allergies anyone has. **Mark them in red!**

* Leave notes for family at home — from you and your HK. Write short notes of encouragement to the HK's siblings. Good luck in your game tonight! Hope your math test goes well! Thanks for cleaning the bathroom! Whatever it might be, there are still things going on in their lives. Even when you are absent they still need to feel your presence.

* Keep all papers together, if possible. Use a BIG three-ring binder with pockets to hold loose items and the small bits of paper you will accumulate — notes, prescriptions, receipts, etc. Clear, top loading, three-ring, sheet covers are perfect for this purpose. You can purchase calculators, zipper pockets (for extra pens/pencils) and other items to personalize your binder and make it more efficient for you.

To save precious time and energy, put things back where they belong — each time — in their place. An accordion file or color-coded files for each category is helpful with all the paperwork. Also, have someone help

Helps & Hope

Also, have someone help you organize the papers and assist you if needed. Sometimes you need that "second brain."

you organize the papers and assist you if needed. Sometimes you need that "second brain" to think through situations with dividers or a box with dividers. Your big notebook is separate from the HUGE notebook you may have received from the staff when your HK was first admitted.

Helps & Hope

Refuge in God

*The eternal God is your refuge,
And underneath are the
everlasting arms....*
— Deuteronomy 33:27a

Get baskets or containers to hold many of the items you and your child need at the hospital for quick and easy transport from home to hospital...to home...as you chalk up *frequent flyer mileage*.

The demanding heart journey requires stamina. As you make the hospital environment more pleasant, you nurture your child and yourself. In the next chapter, more words of encouragement and information strengthen you on your journey.

✳

The LORD [is] my shepherd; I shall not want.
He makes me to lie down in green pastures;
He leads me beside the still waters.
Psalm 23:1-2

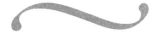

A crisis doesn't come in a vacuum.
But it does come in clumps.

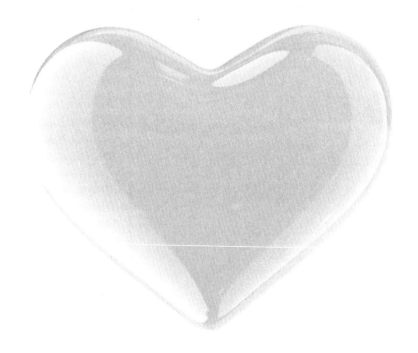

Chapter Six

Forewarned is Forearmed

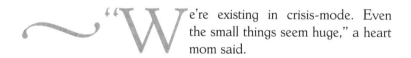"We're existing in crisis-mode. Even the small things seem huge," a heart mom said.

Two Sides of a Crisis

We think of "crisis" as only a negative thing, but the Chinese use two characters with two opposite meanings for crisis. One represents "danger," and the other, "opportunity" (opportunity for growth). Both are valid.

If families view a crisis totally as "danger," dysfunction sets in. Because of the severe distress, they're unable to discover and appreciate resources from within the family and end up fragmented. They blame family members (and anyone else involved), prohibit the sharing of feelings, deny what is happening, and stick to rigid

59

decisions. We do what we've learned to do.

However, when a crisis is also viewed as "opportunity," positive growth occurs and the family remains functional. They face the reality of the situation, but choose not to be thrown by it. Each family member is encouraged to share their feelings, as they draw upon resources (strengths) already in the family, and figure out how to get what is needed to make the best decisions.

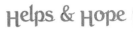

Helps & Hope

Strength to accomplish simple daily tasks may be siphoned when we only think of the crisis as a "danger."

Two Types of Crisis

A *developmental crisis* may seem huge at the time for some; child goes to kindergarten, son gets driver's license, daughter gets married. But these are simply stages in life which many people experience, compared to an *acute crisis* (such as your heart journey). An acute crisis hastens the process of change and hurls families into changing roles, responsibilities, routines, and life-styles (economics).

"As I flipped through the stack of bills, it hit. I thought the regular bills were huge — it's nothing compared to this new medical stack. I wish I'd appreciated how easy life *was*."

All family members begin a "grief" process — giving up dreams of a more perfect life.

Family Patterns

The family is more than the sum of individual family members, but also how they relate, communicate, and solve problems.

Families develop unique patterns of response to crises as they deal with day-to-day life — who has the right to make decisions; how differ-

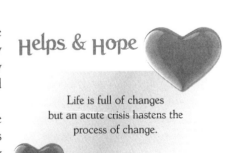

Helps & Hope

Life is full of changes but an acute crisis hastens the process of change.

ences of opinion are handled; and how emotions can/ should be expressed. Some family patterns are constructive while other patterns are destructive. Much depends on on-going issues not addressed before the acute crisis struck. The outcome may de-

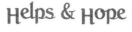

Helps & Hope

The family is more than the sum of individual family members

pend on the willingness of family members to be flexible in the "new normal" of this journey.

✻ A family needs flexibility to cope in crises — to bend during the storms, but not to break. One of the most challenging times deals with parent-teen issues. Adolescence means change. That's growing up — changing. The parent must be flexible (look at the good parts). Be secure and mature (you are the adult), listen not lecture, allow the teen room and space, speak in a calm and affirming voice, keep a good sense of humor — and try to look at teen years as a great "adventure." Remember, this too shall pass.

✻ A rigid family has just one response to crisis and when that fails, they fall apart — can't adapt. Change upends them.

Families develop a particular closeness/distance barometer.

✻ Too close: "Your family can't *be* too close," a mom said. The problem arises when individuals in the family can't identify with their own feelings and can't think of self — just the family. Some (especially the one who does the most) can turn into a martyr. "Why doesn't my husband just help without being asked?" Individuals in the family who are overly dependent on each other don't develop the strength needed to handle crises alone — and crises are a part of life.

✻ Too distant: Individuals in the family, who keep their distance from each other, may appear cold, indifferent, and lack communication skills. They're not hostile, but express neither positive nor negative feelings towards each other. They don't have emotional support from their family — as everyone turns inward.

Family functioning before the crisis — whether it be too close or distant, with some work, can change a negative outcome to a positive one. Slow down and connect with each other on this heart journey. Again, the family is more than the sum of individual family members — but all are needed.

Question/Answer: What is your family like?

Family Reactions

Because family reactions are complex, the following ways empower and enable families to better deal with crises.

Crises trigger disturbing (strong) emotions. Anxiety, guilt, regret, and anger catch us by surprise as they shoot to the surface. These are frightening and uncomfortable, and usually followed by guilt. Thoughts are plagued by what you failed to say, or did you say too much? "I can't believe I'm mad at that person (child or family member). And I'm mad at God for allowing this." Then you're angry at yourself for feeling angry, and the cycle of negative feelings continues *fueled by the fear of the unknown.*

✳ Some families have a rule (spoken or unspoken) that they are not to feel angry, and not to share negative feelings. Some depressed women (and men) stuff their anger, and the spouse doesn't allow her (or him) to express those negative feelings — "Don't be so negative."

✳ Many times, especially a husband wants to take care of his wife and family, and when someone asks, "How are things?" he gives his pat answer, "Okay." He slips into denial and shuts off communication. His wife shuts down and tells others, "Why bother talking to him, he won't let me tell him how I feel anyway." Since they haven't worked through the grief process (whatever the crisis is), they may fill their time staying busy...busy...busy — and don't have "time" to talk.

Crises alter communication patterns. The family may depend on a certain member as the link in receiving and sharing information. If that person is sick or can't fulfill this role, patterns of communication are altered. Under normal circumstances, the family may be open with communication. But a family in crisis has to decide *how* to communicate; *how* to handle certain information; *how* much to share with other family members. If individuals aren't told what is going on, they may think the situation is worse than it is. They need information to begin their walk through the grief process. "I wish I could only give an update once and not talk about it again," a mom said. "And I never know how much to tell outside the family," a dad added.

Crises cause time pressures and increased fatigue. Everyone is running on empty, time to recoup is limited, and none of us make great decisions when we're exhausted. **Take the time to recoup and regroup. Remember, this isn't a sprint, it's a marathon**.

Some families may function well in crisis-mode, which becomes their comfort zone, but when the crisis subsides, they fall apart — or slowly drift apart. They kept occupied dealing with all the variables and didn't address their on-going issues which were there before the crisis.

Question/Answer: What is your family like?

Healthy Ways Families Deal with Stress

Not all stressors are huge like your child's heart defect. Keep your eyes open for the smaller stressors that hurl you against the wall, "What's the matter with me? I'm bawling because

I can't find my keys." Remember that pile of stress we've been building? Those lost keys are just one more clump to add to the pile.

Identify the stressors realistically; then focus on the positive. Don't get stuck, but work through the problems with a plan. Crises come in continuing clumps.

Bombarded family time and finances continue to pile up. Below are positive strategies for coping.

Self Talk — you are what you think you are. Break the negative talk cycle. You are unique and wonderful. And your child loves you like he or she loves *no one* else. That alone is an amazing affirmation of who you are. Take a look around. No matter how bleak your situation is, there are others' who need your strengths and abilities. Reach out and help someone else — especially others less fortunate than you.

Family Meeting — pull together and discuss what needs to be done (list). How often things to be done, and how to do them. Give choices in what each person wants to do. At times, change roles in who does what, but make sure everyone is on board with the changes. If your family shared responsibilities before the crisis, that is a plus, if not, all will need to learn how to do so now.

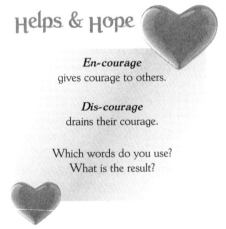

Helps & Hope

En-courage
gives courage to others.

Dis-courage
drains their courage.

Which words do you use?
What is the result?

* Everyone's emotional energy needs to go into helping the solution, not dividing and arguing — which defuses everyone's energy (some don't have much in the first place). This is a team effort with combined strengths like the wagon teams struggling through hardships pushing west. Each person had responsibilities and desperately needed each other as they dealt with daily crises. *This very crisis (the heart journey) may help your family learn to grow together through feelings of accomplishment.*

✱ Communication, whether good or bad, is the process through which we relate to others. Open and clear communication is positive and helpful as information, and feelings are shared. It keeps everyone in the loop day-by-day as much as possible. Poor communication shuts down solutions — when someone criticizes, acts superior, or doesn't listen. Conflicts over decisions drain the fragile empty tanks even further, and problems worsen. Some families with "extra baggage" stagger when the new clumps are dumped.

✱ One key to help members pull together is *fairness*. What are their ages and abilities? Does each family member *have a say* in family decisions (set the goals). Family members need to be part of deciding consequences in cases of misconduct or unacceptable behavior. Discuss accountability in advance — another step in helping move the family toward cooperation. This applies in normal times or the new normal(s), brings closeness between family members, and builds up the individuals for now and later. Be careful who carries most of the load — which usually is mom. Chart how the family shares responsibilities during and after the crisis. Keep communication lines open, don't assume everyone will just "get it." There are no mind readers.

✱ Turn down the volume when talking, and watch out for put downs. Show others respect and affirm them.

✱ Plan ahead to spend time every day if possible talking with family members. First, turn off the TV, computer, games, anything that is a physical distraction from people in that room. Mealtimes are

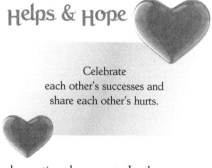

Helps & Hope

Celebrate each other's successes and share each other's hurts.

great for sharing food and emotional support. In the morning, talk about what will happen during their day, and then at dinner, discuss what happened. Celebrate each other's successes and share each other's hurts.

"At mealtime we had each member say something they were thankful for."

When you hear each other's thoughts, it brings joy to everyone. (Endorphins set off). We *reframe* the situation through thankfulness. Once again, a crisis has two sides — danger, and opportunity for growth.

✳ Listen to what the other person is saying. Crisis brings about strong feelings, so let them vent those (catharsis).

"Everyone in our family was a sender, we needed some receivers," a dad said.

"It was like a zoo." The only quiet sibling said, "They didn't notice that I wasn't a sender. Everyone was trying to top the others with stories, and I didn't really fit in — but no one noticed, because I sat there and smiled. I wasn't sure if I was loved during those times."

✳ Be honest, but kind. Speak the truth in love. Avoid manipulating to get your way.

Say what you mean and mean what you say. Be a person of your word — in small and big things.

Question/Answer: What is your family like?

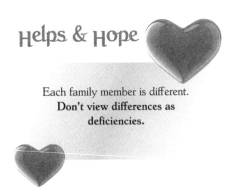

Helps & Hope

Each family member is different.
**Don't view differences as
deficiencies.**

Conclusion

Caregiver, you're riding the waves as they slam on the shoreline boulders. Then you catch your breath as the waves recede and you float on the white foam. In the distance, you spot the next breaker building — but for the present minutes, hours, or days, you rest in the calm.

Let God join you in the calm and the chaos. He's been in both.

But the LORD stood with me and strengthened me...
2 Timothy 4:17

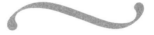

My grace is sufficient for you,
for my power is made perfect in weakness.

— 2 Corinthians 12:9

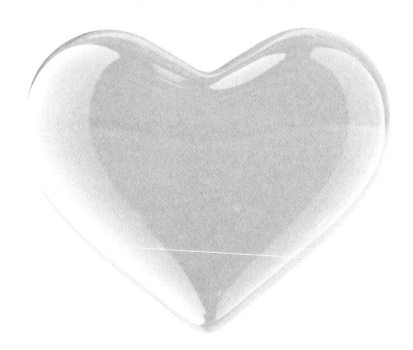

Chapter Seven

Caring for the Caregiver

*S*hould the cabin lose pressure, oxygen masks *will fall from the ceiling in front of you. If you are traveling with small children, place the mask on yourself first, then place a mask on the child.*

For decades, the airline industry has been sharing a valuable life lesson with millions of people. Adults' natural inclination says children first. Period. But how can you help your child if you can't breathe?

With a heart diagnosis comes loss of control, fears for the future, lack of privacy, ravaged routines, and financial worries — and those are just the obvious onslaughts. In the midst of these who takes care of the caregiver? Only the caregiver can add this responsibility to the never-ending list, but they rarely do. Why don't caregivers take care of themselves? Here are some typical responses:

"But I'm not the sick one. I feel guilty even thinking about my needs."

"I hardly have the energy to take care of my HK, much less myself."

"My brain is foggy all the time, so I just wander from one decision to the next."

Helps & Hope

Your child's emotional survival depends on your survival.

These answers all sound valid, but what's the bottom line? If the caregiver goes down the tube, the rest of the family will too. It's hard to recognize this problem when you're in the midst of a crisis, but it's real and moms are often the ones who fall prey to it. We've heard many dads say, "She thinks she's the only one who can do it right." And that is understandable, but what is the outcome?

Lack of Oxygen — Compassion Fatigue

Compassion, of course, is a good thing, but compassion fatigue isn't good for anyone. You care deeply about your child, but you can care too much.

"Care too much? You can't care too much," one mom said. "I just can't leave my child's side — ever. I'm getting sleep; fifteen minutes at a time adds up. Okay, so I'm also snacking, but I'm really not hungry. You don't understand. I have to be here 24/7, and I'm sorry, but no one else can do this. This is my whole life."

But there is a price: fatigue. Compassion fatigue drains precious energy, and it is not a respecter of persons. It's an equal opportunity problem that can attack parents, family, doctors, nurses — all the people in your child's life. Caring and sympathy are good things, just counterproductive when taken to the extreme.

To relieve compassion fatigue and provide yourself with a bit of caretaking, do your best to connect with yourself, with others, and with God on a regular basis. These connections are vital

Helps & Hope

If the caregiver goes down the tube, the rest of the family will too.

to give you strength to continue the journey. They act like a shot of endorphins and they'll help you take better care of your HK. This chapter looks at ways to make these connections within the framework of your overwhelmed, fatigued life.

Helps & Hope

Forgetfulness is Okay

"But I'm sure I won't forget."
Yes, you will.
It can be expected.

Keep Your Oxygen Mask On

✱ Value time — life is precious, even when you're struggling for breath, juggling meetings and clinic appointments away from work, negotiating endlessly with insurance companies and HMOs, feeling totally alone while encircled by doctors, residents, nurses, interns, nurses aids, technicians in your child's hospital room. All are there to help your child — still, you feel alone. Helpless.

Each day is a gift. Find things to celebrate, even simple things each day. Write a Thanks-giving list, and the endorphins will kick in. You act better, then feel better. Actions come before feelings.

My friend, Lisa Kay Hauser is a fellow author, and a CHD mom. She says, "If you want to feel better, choose joy! There's so much we can be joyful about. Yes, there are also those things that kick us down, but we don't have to 'live there.' We can choose to live joyfully, instead, regardless of our circumstances. It only takes a moment to look around and find something to appreciate: the lab tech that always smiles; the cup of coffee you shared with your spouse this morning; catching your child making silly faces at herself in the mirror. She's an HK, but she still knows how to be silly. Life is still good. Living joyfully is a choice — even in the most difficult times."

Don't let the calendar dictate special occasions. Place a calendar on your wall (home or hospital) and have each family member write at least one thing a day that they were thankful for — the sun shining, they can hear, have AC or heat in home, family together. Many times, the younger the child is, the more heartfelt the thanks.

✳ Small but significant. It's very, very easy to focus on the emergencies, prescriptions, and relapses — but also focus on the squeeze your mom gave your hand, the funny story the nurse told you — all just as real as the pain felt. The hand squeeze or story was small but significant.

✳ Let go of other's burdens — you can't solve everyone's problems — don't even try. Experience breeds personal growth and power. It's okay to "mother" but don't smother. Especially true with teens as the hormones hit with independence in tow. "Why does my mom keep worrying about me?"

✳ Beware of those who attempt to rip off your oxygen mask. Most won't do that on purpose, but set your boundaries. Don't give in to guilt, "You're going to dinner with your husband — and leaving Jason at the hospital, by himself?" "You're so strong. I could never do what you do." You want to scream, *No, I'm not strong, and I'd like someone else to be.* Refer to You-niquely Made Personalities (Appendix One).

✳ Stop denying you are exhausted. Ask for help. Yes, you do know your child better than anyone and can read his/her body language. And yes, you know what they want and how they want it. And yes, you've heard everything the doctors have said, and googled any related information on your child's disease. However, you can't be everything for your child. Stop, slap that mask back on, take a deep breath, and ask for help.

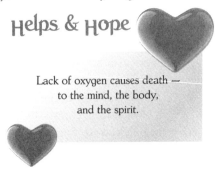

Helps & Hope

Lack of oxygen causes death — to the mind, the body, and the spirit.

Asking for help does a lot to forge connections with family and friends. No one can read your mind. You'll have needs your family and friends have never thought about unless they've been on this journey. And, even if they have, all situations are different.

If you've had to be "the strong one," it will be difficult to ask for help. Remember, this isn't about you; this is about quality time for your HK — which is enhanced if you've asked for help.

When friends say, "How can I help?" **tell** them. They wouldn't ask unless they were willing. While your child is having a treatment, or napping, grab your notebook and jot down a few specific things that you can turn over to friends — from cleaning your house, bringing meals, and watching the siblings, to simply coming and sitting with you to talk — and to let you catch a quick shower.

"Showers have never felt so good," most moms say.

Your focus is on your sick child, but there are others in your peripheral vision. Let them into your life, to help you, your child, and allow them to be part of the solution. They want to be there for you. It will be a blessing for all of you.

* Keep your sense of identity. You aren't just *Jasonsmom* or *Chelseysdad*. You aren't just a *heartmom*. You are you — a special person who is the mom of Jason — the dad of Chelsey, who has a heart defect.

Connecting with Self
Plan Ahead

One of the most important ways to connect with yourself is to plan ahead with your calendar and notebook/ journal. Your mind is crammed with schedules, tests, protocols, when and where sibs need to be, the people who are dropping off food for your family tonight (always a good thing), and the fact that your house is a wreck (which feels like a bad thing). In the middle of juggling all those thoughts in your head, you might think, "Did I call Susan back yesterday?" On it goes.

Now is the time to slow down. Take a take a deep breath. Grab your pen, and write out everything that you need to do. If you're still feeling overwhelmed, prioritize the list. Remember that you can pass some of these things to your friends and come-alongsiders. Put their names beside those items, (i.e. Ask

Helps & Hope

God, grant me the serenity to accept the things I cannot change, courage to change the things I can, and wisdom to know the difference.
— Reinhold Neibuhr

Darlene to pick up Joey from soccer practice on Thursday; Ask Rosemary about picking up dry cleaning at Joe's on 11th street).

Rank the tasks in the order of importance to be done. Read it every night and every morning, and check off what you've accomplished. Prioritize what needs to be done for the next day. The notebook may become your new best friend. It will tell you what to do, and when it needs doing. You won't waste precious energy trying to remember whatever you were supposed to remember. Keep the notebook with you and several pens and pencils with it. Pens and pencils mysteriously disappear when you need them, so plan ahead. For a dollar you can get a pack of eight pens at most stores.

Still overwhelmed by the uncontrollable situation? Pray the words written by Reinhold Neibuhr, "God, grant me the serenity to accept the things I cannot change, courage to change the things I can, and wisdom to know the difference."

Paste that simple, yet, powerful prayer on the inside of your binder if you have to so that you see those words often to remind you that you DON'T have control over the universe and that's okay. That really is the way it's supposed to be.

Jumpstart the Positive Messengers

Stress sends out a barrage of negative messengers (adrenaline and cortisol in particular) in the brain, throwing us into fight-or-flight mode. We may overly react in anger or run away from the problem. To combat stress, we have to *choose* to jumpstart the positive messengers — endorphins.

Endorphin is a substance in the brain that attaches to the same cell receptors that morphine does. It abolishes the sensation of pain. The brain doesn't know if the person is really happy, it just responds to the happy messengers.

Result? We feel better.

Endorphins are needed in all phases of life to help our physical and emotional

Helps & Hope

Ability

List the things you can change, and then tackle the list one at a time. Put the rest on the back burner.

states. They also boost the immune system. Fortunately, we can add some activities into our daily routine (or lack thereof) to release those precious endorphins. Let's look at ways to do that.

Laughter

"I don't think I'll ever be able to laugh again," a mom said.

Then another mom added, "One day I caught myself laughing at something on TV and I felt guilty. My kids were relieved to hear me laugh, and it opened a discussion about our new normal, which had little laughter. We all seemed to need permission to laugh."

Laughter (inside jogging) oxygenates your entire body, which is desperately needed during stressful times. Is your blood pressure up? Depression and tension setting in? Having trouble digesting your food? Try a dose of laughter!

Sometimes we'd like someone else to initiate our laughter. We'd like to have someone tickle us, or tell a joke — then we'd totally laugh our head off and not think of anything but laughing and gasping for air! But that's probably not going to happen, so you'll need to take matters into your own hands.

Now, what's funny to you? Watch a slapstick movie, read a humorous book, or listen to a ridiculous CD. Find a five-year-old and have him tell you a knock-knock joke — then watch him bend over with laughter. It's contagious.

Sleep

Sleep is another powerful way to release endorphins. To refresh your body, you need six to eight hours sleep. REM sleep (rapid eye movement) occurs during the last few hours when you're dreaming.

The early hours give rest for the body, but the later hours renew and rebuild it. This recommendation may seem impossible knowing how hard it is to get the sleep needed.

One dad said, "It seems weird. You're so tired, you'd think you'd fall asleep and stay asleep. But being that exhausted, you can't fall asleep, and then you toss and turn. Or, if you do fall asleep, you wake up in the middle of the night. Your mind races, and you can't go back to sleep. It's really strange."

Whether you're in the hospital room, at home, staying in the Ronald McDonald house, or wherever you're trying to rest, attempt to get eight hours of sleep — even if it's interrupted. You also may need to switch off occasionally with a family member or friend and have them spend the night with your child. Results? You have a fresh viewpoint in the morning as your body, mind, and emotions are renewed. You need that REM sleep for the long haul.

Why do you cuddle your sleeping child? Because you want them to feel comfortable, serene, and secure. And you'll do whatever it takes to make that happen. That's how God feels when He watches any of His children sleep. He wants you comfortable and serene — secure in His arms.

Sheets and pillowcases wad into wrinkles during fitful sleep. Turning the pillow over to the cool side relieves the heat and moisture from your face. After flipping the pillow, nestle in, and thank Him for His care. Eight hours (even interrupted) is ideal, but some nights you'll get little or no sleep and fall asleep in the middle of the day.

Try to schedule a power nap between various visitors and staff coming and going. Dim the lights, and curl up with your blankie. Set a quiet alarm for fifteen to thirty minutes. You'll probably wake up groggy, but that goes away and you'll have a surge of energy to carry you through the evening.

Exercise

Exercise is another way to release endorphins. You may be thinking, "Oh yeah, when is that supposed to happen?" Time is indeed a problem, but we're not talking about a full workout here. Walk laps up and down the hospital hall, take the stairs to the cafeteria, or pump iron (two

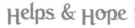

eight-ounce cans of food will do). It doesn't take much because anything helps. Ten minutes of walking gets your blood flowing. It needs the help. Ten minutes three times a day is fantastic. The family room on your floor may have a treadmill. Take advantage of it. If you're at home and your children are old enough to leave for a few minutes, walk up and down your block. If they're not old enough, then walk in your house and turn up your favorite "walking" music. If you have a treadmill at home, that's even better exercise to keep the blood flowing.

There's an added benefit while you're in the hospital: walking requires leaving the room. This may be very difficult for mom, but it's needed. Pace yourself. Again, this journey is a marathon, not a short run. By taking even ten minutes to exercise, you aren't just caring for yourself — you're doing the best thing for everyone else too.

Sunshine

Open those blinds and turn on lots of lamps. Light increases your level of serotonin, a hormone that helps elevate your mood and decrease fatigue. On this journey you definitely want some serotonin to give you more energy and courage to face the day.

However, the amount of light your child can tolerate depends on your HK's condition, so check with the nurse first.

Deep Breaths

Bring oxygen deep down into your lungs through your nose, count to five, and then breathe out through your mouth. As you breathe out you release toxins from your body. Repeat ten times, three times a day. This clears your brain, burns calories, and relaxes the body. It's free. What more can you ask?

Also, drink lots of water. "Drink water? But it doesn't have caffeine!"

As stress bombards your body, toxins (poisons) are building. Deep breaths release toxins from your body and water flushes them out. (Yes, that means frequenting the bathroom.) Try to get eight ounces, six times a day. Keep filling that water bottle.

Helps & Hope

The Journey

Pace yourself. This journey is a marathon, not a short run.

Food

Food also has a powerful effect on the way we feel, and stress can have a profound impact on the way we eat. "I'm just not hungry," one mom said. And her friend replied, "I just eat all the time."

Where's the balance?

A mom's advice, "You talk about a vicious cycle. You're exhausted, then you overdose on caffeine and sugar to keep you awake at night to check on things. When you come down off the caffeine and sugar you get depressed, so you hit those foods and drinks again. Smart, huh? Well, we know it's a crutch, but those long hours, either in the hospital or at home — it just happens. Try to watch what and when you're eating. You don't even realize it until you look at all the empty cans, Styrofoam containers, and cookie wrappers."

If you keep a journal, take notes not only of what your HK is eating and drinking, but you too. Your body has got to be the best it can be for everyone's sake.

Connecting with Others

"I never thought I'd ever shut people out of my life, but as I've become wearier, that's what I've done," said a mom. "I know others really care, but I don't have the strength at times to talk. How can I explain things over and over and over..."

Internet and E-Mail

It can be overwhelming to try to stay connected to all your loved ones and all the people who care about your child. Check into the websites Caringbridge (www.caringbridge.com), Carepages (www. carepages.com), or CareFlash.com (www.careflash.com) for free, personal, easy-to-create web pages that help you connect with friends and family (see Resource Three).

You can create a page for your child and post regular updates. This will allow friends and family to stay connected to your family at a time when you may have little time for phone calls. You may want to keep the site updated yourself, but there may be days (or nights) when you can't. You may also choose to have someone else keep up the site for you. However, many parents find when they e-mail others or post to a personal website, it's an outlet for their emotions — a catharsis. And of course, it's a blessing to read the e-mails or posts made in response. Those prayers and encouraging words will lift you up and your child. Communication goes both ways.

In Person

Although there's great value in connecting with others, it can also be difficult to do so. You're living a reality most people will never experience. When bombarded with too many inquiries about how you're doing, just muster a slight smile and say, "We're exhausted, but thank you for asking."

You'll never have the time or ability to completely explain your new life to them. If you're a more introverted Blue or Green personality, dealing with other people wears you out. To be re-filled you need your quiet space and time. To set your boundaries with others, rehearse what you will say and thank them for their thoughtfulness. Have an outgoing Yellow family member or friend be the contact person for you. It will give you the space you need to regroup and will use your Yellow friend's strengths, which will bring her joy interacting with others and sharing some of your load.

Do you want to be kept in the loop with friends? You've probably forgotten there is a loop — the outside world, your former life before heart defects.

Have friends keep you up-to-date on what's going on, but beware. When they tell you about the outside world, they'll talk about their lives — their lives with healthy children, no clinics, no pain. You may end up feeling like this mom: "I want to hear, but I get jealous when I think what their kids can do and mine can't."

Another mom said, "I *love* my friends. I mean, I *really* do, but their "big issues" are so... *trivial*. We are dealing with life and death issues, and they are griping about carpool and coupons. I just want to scream. Then, of course, I feel terrible for feeling that way because before our baby was born with CHD, carpool was one of my big issues, too. And, *at the time*, it seemed huge."

Pray for an open heart to listen to others. Those parents don't know what to say to you; you be their guide. You need them, and they need to hear from you.

While it's important to maintain your connections with those in the outside world, it's also valuable to reach out to those inside your new world. You need those other foggy-brained families wandering around the hospital, in the clinics, and at support groups and camps.

You may think, "But I've only begun this journey; some have been on it a long time." Everyone has something to add to the other's journey. Remember, you're their best resource and know how they feel as few others do.

Connecting with God

It's easy to see that you can connect inwardly with yourself and horizontally with others. But you can also connect vertically with God. He constantly reaches out to you. Each of us is uniquely touched by Him. Gary Chapman's book, *The Five Love Languages*, (Resource One) discusses the way humans interact and love one another — and to understand connecting with God more fully, read Chapman's book *The Five Love Languages of God*. As 1 John 4:19 says, "We love [God], because he first loved us."

Talk and Listen to Him

You may feel as if your life has been struck by continuous waves as you lie weary on the beach. But you're not alone. God the

Father is always there ready to help, but you need to talk to Him, and listen for His answers.

Helps & Hope

The Bible is more real than the book you are holding in your hands.
— Brennan Manning

"When our baby daughter was going through so many surgeries and in pain, the Lord kept bringing scriptures to me in the Psalms that gave me what I needed — I needed to be still. Psalm 46:10, 'Be still and know that I am God,' He kept saying, 'Be still, wait, listen.' And there was one, Ecclesiastes 2:17 that I could really relate to growing up on a ranch in Oklahoma where the wind blows all the time, '...all (life) of it is meaningless, a *chasing after the wind*.' That's what I'd done in my life — chasing after the wind. His words carried me through those dark days, and it (that scripture) still speaks to my heart today," said Gregg.

Journal

Helps & Hope

Whether writing by hand or using a computer, it's amazing to keep track of God's work in your life, especially on this journey. If you don't have a journal, a simple pad of paper will do. Be honest in your feelings. God is not offended — or surprised. Is the new normal still smothering you? Pick the petals off a daisy, but change the words:

Focus not just on the unfairness and problems of life, but also on all that does turn out well. Review the good things of the past, and don't forget in the darkness what you've learned in the light.
— Phillip Yancey

"He loves me, He loves me, He loves me...."

Yes, He does. You'll realize this more and more as you count your blessings. Count them first thing in the morning as you struggle out of bed and the last thing at night as you collapse into it. Count them while you sit on the sofa or scrunched close to your child in the hospital's single bed. Try it during the night as you smack the beeping IV button. You do have blessings, but probably can't remember them because your mind is crammed with the new normal. Take time to think about it, and write them down when you have a chance. If you're thinking, "Blessings? What blessings?" we have some suggestions from fellow travelers.

* "I can see with both eyes. It's that simple; something I took for granted, then I had a problem with my eye and realized how important that was."

* "Being able to get this kind of special care and treatment for my child. In my home country, he would have died."

* "Strangers, who smile at me in the elevator even when I'm standing there in my grubby clothes and I haven't put on makeup."

* "Cafeteria food. Even though I'm sick of eating the same things, it is downstairs."

* "Pinks of sunrise. I've seen lots of them, and they bring hope for a new day after a long dark night. They're especially beautiful as a backdrop for black silhouetted trees."

* "Knowing I can count on others to pray for us. They really care."

Start your own "Thanks-giving" list. Read it over every morning as you wake. God will plant new patterns of thinking (thanks-giving) in your brain. After all, He's your Spiritual Caregiver who never becomes weary of giving care.

Communicate through Music

Music stirs our heartstrings, and surfaces our emotions. Open a Bible to the middle. There you'll find King David's songs from his heart — the Psalms. They're still touching hearts today — our hearts and the heart of God. Long ago, David said,

"The LORD *is* my strength and my shield;
My heart trusted in Him, and I am helped;
Therefore my heart greatly rejoices,
And with my song I will praise Him."

— Psalm 28:7

Blessings continue each day — just keep your eyes on Him.

Tunes and beats change from one generation to the next, but they still connect people to God. Don't hesitate to do that.

Appreciate His Creation

Ever notice how most of the world is either blue or green? Blue water covers most of our globe. Blue skies arch from horizon to horizon, and green vegetation sprouts in trees and grasses. Why so much blue and green? They're calm, cool colors. God knew we would need a majority of calm colors in our hectic lives with occasional splashes of bright reds, yellows, and other colors in the spectrum.

"The heavens declare the glory of God; And the firmament shows His handiwork," Psalm 19:1 says.

Don't miss a day appreciating His handiwork. Early morning or evening, step outside or peek through a window at the rising and setting of the sun—as pinkish-orange rays begin or end a day in your life. Familiarity creeps in as the majesty of our created world becomes humdrum. We take it for granted because we see it every day. Ask God for a fresh viewpoint, then gaze at whatever creation is nearby. Look closely at any flower—the colors in any flower always blend. The hues compliment each other and never clash. Another one of the Creator's coincidences.

Over two thousand years ago, Jesus spoke to crowds on a hillside. He told them not to worry, because they couldn't add a single hour to their lives. Then he added not to even worry about clothes. "...Consider the lilies of the field, how they grow: they neither toil nor spin; and yet I say to you that even Solomon in all his glory was not arrayed like one of these." (Matthew 6:26-29).

He is the Creator of everything created. Connect with Him.

Above all, trust Him.

That is how to truly connect with Him. He's in control of all things—even your circumstances. Earlier in the book I talked about the tunnel of life with a sick child, I quoted Isaiah 43:2 "When you pass through the waters, I will be with you. And through the rivers, they shall not overflow you...." Don't miss that word "through." It is very important. Some paths are so difficult and dark that no way out can be seen. You appear to be walking in a cave and the further you travel the darker it gets. But you are not in a cave but a tunnel. True faith will always see a vision of a sovereign, faithful God and be strengthened, not shattered. The one who trusts in God can be sure, even in the darkest tunnels of life that God knows our path and He will bring us through.

Jesus Christ, God's Son walked the darkest of paths to save us, and He says to everyone for whom the burden is too great, "Come unto me all ye that are weary and heavy laden and I will give you rest. For my yoke is easy and my burden is light."

He did not promise life without burdens but He promised that if we come to Him, if we trust Him, if we lean everything on Him, He will give us rest. He will lead us through every tunnel, even the final one. Connect with him.

Now connect with family as you fly with your flock in the next chapter. Everyone in your flock needs encouragement for the long flight as their weary wings flap, buffeted by storm clouds.

My flesh and my heart fail;
[But] God is the strength of my heart and my portion forever.
Psalm 73:26

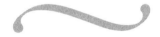

You don't really understand human nature
unless you know why a child on a merry-go-round
will wave at his parents every time around —
and why his parents will always wave back.

— **William D. Tammeus**

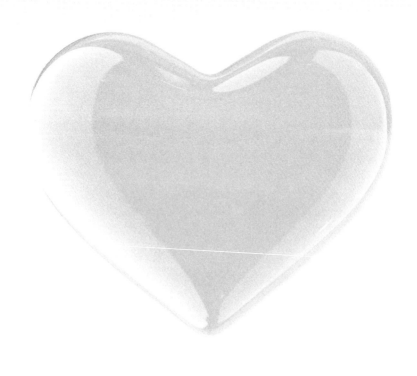

Chapter Eight

Family Flocks

et's consider some lessons from the wobbly V. You hear them before you see them. Suddenly, they swoosh overhead, the wobbly V of Canada geese gliding across the horizon, honking encouragement to one another for their extensive journey.

Heart families endure long journeys too, and desperately need encouragement. Surprisingly perhaps, we can learn from flocks of flying geese. Let these lessons strengthen your weary wings.

In a flock of geese flying in V formation, the lead goose rotates back in the formation when it grows tired. Are you the lead goose? Are you the main caregiver on the heart journey? If so, you may feel you can never rotate back and must take the lead, 24/7. Besides, what would others think if you weren't there all the time?

The fact is, dear lead goose, you are on an extremely long journey. Take the opportunity to rotate back at times. Others will need you for the extensive journey. Canada geese work together as they migrate. Each bird in the V flaps its wings, creating an uplift for the following bird, thereby traveling 71 percent further than if each bird flew on its own, as all head in the same direction. Heart families,

too, need to uplift each other for their extensive journey. And the flock needs to fly in the same direction. There are a number of ways to make that happen. Your child doesn't need to hear conflicting advice.

For example, Mom may say, "He needs more rest."

Dad may respond, "No, he needs to get out of that bed."

Do your best to communicate your ideas and listen to others' opinions. If you do disagree about strategies for your child, discuss the differences of opinion in private.

Each goose's special cadence "Honk!" inspires courage. "Keep on going! You can do it!"

However, if a goose has to drop out of formation, another goose (or two) drops out and flies alongside him. If he lands to recoup, the other two stay with him until they can all rejoin the flock. In the same way, each family member inspires courage with special words and actions to "Keep on going! You can do it!" However, there may be times when a family member needs to drop out of formation with the flock. This may be due to health, emotional overload, or other hindering circumstances. Others (immediate or extended family) need to be aware and come alongside until that member is able to join the flock again.

Understandably, most of the family's attention is directed toward the heart child, so keep your eyes open for others who may need help. In the darkness, geese continue to communicate by honking, so no goose gets lost. By effective communication, talking and listening to each other, no one in the family gets lost in the darkness, and all stay connected.

Your family may have had great coping skills in the past; if so, those skills will probably help you. However, this is an entirely new journey. Unlike geese that follow the same migration path year after year, you and your flock have not traveled this way before. Individuals' thoughts on issues may change daily — even hourly — so take time each day to share those feelings. Holding them in is counterproductive, but remember to share them in love.

In your flock, a united front may be divided over finances, rules for siblings at home, even parents' faith. "I know God will heal him," a father may say about his son. That rings hollow to the spouse who chides, "This is the real world of heart defects we're dealing with." Be patient and tolerant of your differences. Again, they make sense to the other person.

Another part of your life that needs attention is your sexual relationship.

"But I feel guilty seeking pleasure in the midst of all this," a mom said.

"Besides, I'm too exhausted." a dad added, "And I'm worn down worrying about finances. I never even have time to shave. I look perpetually stubbly."

Plan ahead and take the time needed to stay close and reassured of each other's love.

Generations Fly Alongside

"I don't know what I would have done without my mother," said the young woman holding her toddler. "I know it's killing her watching all this, but she's been a rock."

"Grandparents put lots of miles on their vehicles transporting the siblings when we've needed help, or when school drop off and pick up times have not coordinated with medical appointments," a mom said.

You may or may not have help from your parents. If you do, you may not view some things they say and do as a help.

How do grandparents come alongside without taking over? It isn't easy. They not only worry about their grandchild, but also their child — two generations of worrying you'd call it. Their emotional tanks have emptied also. Many emotional and interpersonal issues come to the surface on this journey. As the generations try to work together, things can get tough. Some parents have voiced these feelings:

Helps & Hope

One of life's greatest mysteries is how the boy who wasn't good enough to marry your daughter can be the father of the smartest grandchild in the world.

* "I'm glad Mom and Dad are here, but..."

* "They make me feel inadequate, second-guessing my decisions."

* "They sigh all the time — especially around their grandson." (Review the Blue personality who feel others' pain deeply.)

* "They instruct the nurses and anyone else who walks in the room on how they should do their job." (Review Red personality who makes sure everything is done right.)

* "I guess the bottom line is that all the old bad things (memories) rise to the top, and I can't deal with those and the new bad things."

If any of these thoughts ring true, now is the time to confront lovingly. You may be surprised at unspoken thoughts lodged in your parents' minds as everyone continues reeling. Plan ahead what you want to say to them, where to say it, and, most importantly, how to say it.

What to say? Here are a few brief ideas:

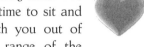

* "Mom and Dad, thanks so much for your support. We're really going to need it for the long haul. We need a time to sit and talk with you out of hearing range of the

It's funny that those things your kids did that got on your nerves seem so cute when your grandchildren do them.

children, because we're all running on empty emotionally, and we need to have a game plan."

* "(Child's name) needs all of us to be on the same page dealing with his medical care. He needs us to be as positive as possible because he can read our body language. Smiles are necessary, and we have to watch the sighing. Actually, this is true for all our children. We're all in this together, and we may need to touch base like this each day for a while."

* Where do you say it? Away from the children. How do you say it? Respectfully.

The Rest of the Flock

Probably many of your child's aunts, uncles, and cousins are chiming in, "We're here for you."

Whether they're near or far, keep them in the loop, through e-mail and calls. One person may be the point person to contact the others. Whoever is in your flock, refer to the You-nique-ly Made Personality Study in Resource One for a refresher on your gene pool. Remember, Reds will direct family and staff, Blues will sigh and straighten the room (let them), Yellows will talk constantly to other families and staff (but probably won't remember their names), and Greens will sit for hours lending a listening ear to anyone who needs it. Appreciate each member of your flock.

Flying Through the Holidays

All the holidays can be difficult in the new normal. Roller-coaster emotions soar and dive as families remember previous holidays, struggle through the current one, and anticipate the next ones. Emotions are stretched to the limit. Especially around the holidays, you may find yourself feeling like this mom: "One day we feel blessed, and the next blasted. I'm praying for a balance. Only God can give that, because we can't ourselves."

New Year's

The new normal brings a different perspective on New Year's resolutions. Losing a few pounds or giving up a bad habit pale in comparison to your new life. Looking at January of the new year, you're struck with the preciousness of life, health (in whatever condition that may be), and hopefulness for the future. January 1st pushes you forward.

Plan ahead. Flip the calendar to the upcoming months and write something special to do for someone once a month or more frequently if you can. It may be very small in your sight, but not in God's. Pray for His guidance through each of the 365 days.

Easter

"There can be no permanent loss in the life of My children, for out of the seeds of every calamity rises a whole crop of new victories. It is the way I have made it. The greatest evidence of this truth is Calvary. Out of the cruelty of men with wicked hearts, Christ was made a martyr — but by the Hand of a greater power, He was made to become a Savior — *even the Savior of the very men who put Him to death.*"

~ Frances J. Roberts, *Come Away My Beloved, The Intimate Devotional Classic*

Mother's Day — Healing My Heart

When I knew my baby was fatally ill, I realized the best way to get through the pain of Mother's Day was to comfort others.

It was literally the Mother's Day of a lifetime. The only Mother's Day I would have with my daughter, Hope. She was five months old and because she was born with a metabolic disorder called

Zellweger Syndrome, she was expected to live less than six months. So every day was a gift. And I wanted to enjoy the gift of having her for this Mother's Day rather than focus on the reality that it would be our only one together, which it was.

But perhaps the greatest gift I received was having my eyes opened to the hurting people around me on what, for many, is a very difficult day.

As that day approached, I anticipated the mixture of joy and pain the day would bring. I began to think of people around me — people I knew who had lost their mothers that year and were facing the first Mother's Day without them, those who had lost children and felt the void especially on that day, those I had come in contact with who, like me, had children who would not live until the next Mother's Day, even those who have never been able to conceive or carry a child successfully.

So I made a list and went to the store to buy Mother's Day cards. Now with all the Mother's Day cards on the rack, it is not easy to find a big selection of cards for men who've lost their mothers or mothers who've lost children, so I had to improvise. But I sent out a big stack of cards that year and every year since.

Some people I didn't send cards to. Early Mother's Day morning, I called a woman in my church who had buried her mother who died of breast cancer the month before. I didn't really know her that well and felt a little awkward calling so early on Sunday, but because I reached out to her that difficult day, we became friends for life. Then at church that morning, I looked over and saw a woman with four small children whose husband had recently left her. I walked over and wished her happy Mother's Day, telling her that I thought she was an incredible mother to her children. It seemed to matter.

There's something good that happens to me when I'm able to get my eyes off of my own pain and minister out of it to other people who are hurting. It brings a healing to my heart that could not be found any other way.

I've already begun making my list for this year — the woman in our church whose son took his own life, the husband who is doing his best to parent four children and usher them through the grief of losing their mom in an accident, the woman who is saying a slow good-bye to her mother who has Alzheimers, my friend who miscarried several months ago. And somehow, in the midst of comforting others, through the power of the Holy Spirit I believe I'll be comforted myself.

Nancy Guthrie is the author of *Holding On to Hope: A Pathway Through Suffering to the Heart of God*; and *The One Year Book of Hope*, a daily devotional for those hurting or grieving. www.nancyguthrie.com.

Helps & Hope

My dad is the boss...
until Grandma comes over.
Then he's just one of us.
~ a child in *Kids Say the Greatest Things about God*

💜 Father's Day

Father's Day — a tie, socks, coffee mug? What to give dad? How about "We need you and appreciate all you do."

Overwhelmed by the heart journey, a dad said, "I'm going back to work. At least I know what to do there."

Mom has probably been the main caregiver for your heart child, and you have tried to hold on to your job (not easy with all the time off needed), and have shuttled between the hospital, home (with siblings), kept others in the loop, and attempted to figure out mom's exhausted moods. You are exhausted also, so take care of yourself — run around the block, watch your favorite team on TV, or whatever fills your emotional tank. Your family depends on you for strength, guidance, and unconditional love. Hang in there, dad. Happy Father's Day.

💜 Thanks Giving on Thanksgiving

"Giving thanks on Thanksgiving? A few years ago, that was easy. We repeated the usual God-is-great-God-is-good-and-we-thank-Him-for-our-food-amen prayer. The table groaned with plates full of food, extended family members crowded around the table,and good health was a given. Giving thanks was easy," a mom said. "This year we spent Thanksgiving in the hospital room and ate off the tray next to my child's bed. Our smaller immediate family sat on our child's bed, on a recliner, and at the foot of the bed/sofa. Some volunteers brought in a Thanksgiving meal for everyone on the floor, so the smells and tastes made it feel like Thanksgiving.

We thought back to that first Thanksgiving and the pilgrims who'd spent two months crossing an ocean rocked by storms and landed in the dead of winter. The rest were weak and wouldn't have made it if the Wampanoag Indians hadn't taught them how to plant, hunt, and survive. They shared a bountiful meal and were thankful for food, friends, and health — the basics.

And there we sat in our child's room and deeply appreciated our food, friends, and staff and volunteers, and the health that we had at that present time — the basics — nothing taken for granted. Our prayer came deep from within, an appreciation of all we had, and to our Lord who gives us our 'daily bread.' We now thank Him for the easy times — and His being with us in the difficult ones."

🤍 Merry Christmas!

"When I was putting away the boxes after last year's Christmas, I wondered if our nine-year-old son Tommy would be with us the next Christmas. It is now the next Christmas, and he is still with us — and we are so thankful for his life. We're also thankful for the gift of life that was given him by some wonderful parents who donated their child's heart for another child to live. I'm overwhelmed with appreciation and sadness as I pray for them on their first Christmas without their child here on earth," Colleen said.

"And we rejoice in the most important miracle and gift ever given, the birth of Christ for which we have been given all HOPE, no matter what our circumstances! With thankful hearts to ALL of you who faithfully walk this journey with us." (From Colleen's Carepage.)

As a heart family, you may have a clearer vision of Christmas than the rest of the world. Carols sung about the midnight sky when angels burst forth on the scene and the way the shepherds froze in fear. The angels had to reassure them, "Fear not...."

Today you may be frozen in fear and need reassuring. But just as the angels proclaimed over two-thousand years ago, "Fear not, for behold we bring you good tidings of great joy," that joy came from heaven to earth in the form of a baby.

Now, what traditions do you have in your family? It can be hard to keep up with Christmas traditions when you're living in the new normal. Consider which ones are most important to your heart child and your other children and maintain those traditions. Think about whether the new normal demands some new traditions — and remember Who the season is about.

The Flocks Have Landed

You're heading home. One mom said, "When we got the word that we'd been discharged, we were so excited. We were headed home! Home to my own bed, and my child in her bed. Home with my family, my routines, my washing machine, my neighbors, my refrigerator, my bathroom.... I was truly excited. Then I remembered what another mom had told me — that the transition to home isn't necessarily easy.

That mom told me, 'I was so glad to be going home, I never thought about the downside. I had to put back all the stuff that made the hospital room home and then clean up what hadn't been done while I'd been gone. And you know what else? I missed the professionals down the hall. Even in a house full of people, I felt all alone.'"

A single mom said, "I second-guessed my child's coughs, fever, everything. I was used to the nurses checking in every few hours. I know I can call the nurse at night, but I feel like I'm doing that too much already, even though they say I'm not. I thought I'd feel relieved to be home, and I am, but at first I felt overwhelmed. It just seemed to be up to me 24/7 to know what to do. Who am I going to ask for help in the middle of the night, my other preschool children? But I really am glad to be home."

When you get home, you not only deal with fear and second guessing, you may miss your new hospital family.

"I miss the families we've met on the floor, and wonder how they are doing. I just need to take the time and call them. And the hospital staff have become some of my best friends. I miss being a part of their lives. Sometimes I just call at three in the afternoon and ask what they're doing. I know that sounds silly, but I still feel connected to them."

It may seem strange that there is an adjustment involved in coming home, but many families find that to be the case. *You're not alone.* You adjust to the downside and deal with settling in, and then you can appreciate the positives. You're home! You've completed another step on the journey. Your new normal continues to unfold, and your family is back under one roof continuing that journey. Your family is glad you're home, especially those siblings.

*Be anxious for nothing, but in everything
by prayer and supplication, with thanksgiving,
let your requests be made known to God...*
Philippians 4:6

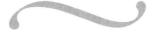

*The highlight of my childhood was making my brother
laugh so hard that food came out his nose.*

— Garrison Keillor, author Lake Woebegone Days

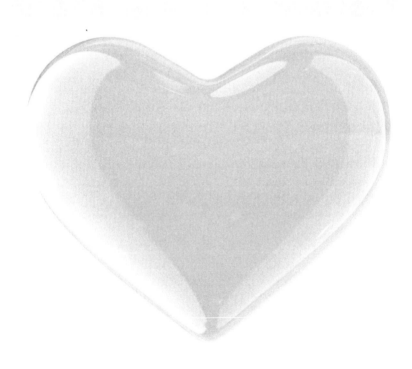

Chapter Nine

Siblings: The Well Ones

There are over 40,000 children diagnosed with heart disease each year in the United States, plus childhood heart survivors. There are at least that many children thrust into the heart arena with them — their siblings — the well ones. Both are victims of heart defects, which affects the rest of their lives. They're on the same road. "But miles apart," a sibling said. We want this chapter to help bring the family closer together.

"You have to take into consideration how you treat the sibling(s) that come after the HK — all the many sonograms done to be sure the fetus is okay. Our daughter had more pictures taken of her 'inside' than she did 'outside' after she was born," a mom said.

Siblings are not small adults; they are children, with childlike perspectives and needs. It's easy to shove a teen sibling into the adult role in your family — but they aren't adults — they just look that way. Siblings, whatever age, communicate in various ways with the HK.

McDonalds:

Overheard from a preschool sibling: *My mommy lives with Ronald McDonald in his house now.*

"I love how grandma explained our son's heart surgery to his three-year-old sibling. 'The doctor will open up that line on his chest and fix his heart.' That seemed to answer her surgery questions quite well."

Siblings are individuals with unique personalities, interests, and their own place in your family's birth order. Siblings need help to cope and carve out their own identity. It's important to be more than just "John's brother."

Most siblings have a healthy heart (HH), but all need love and attention. Parents, do whatever it takes to keep communication open with these siblings. Remember that each of you see things from your own side of the fence.

Let's listen to some viewpoints from the siblings' side of the fence:

❋ "My parents' world is now Kaycy. All the rest of us have to stand in line — way down the line...."

❋ "I keep constantly changing my plans and giving and giving. I don't want to feel jealous, but I do sometimes."

❋ "I feel *invisible*. People just look past or through me, or always just ask about my sister. I'm still here, aren't I?"

Now let's hear from the parents:

❋ "Heart siblings are a wealth of misinformation. I'd never have guessed what they were thinking, not in a million years."

* "I can't meet all their needs. Most of the time, I don't even know what those needs really are. I just live on guilt."

* "As long as the sibling doesn't demand attention, we think everything's okay. I wish that were true."

Opening the Gate

What are the keys to unlocking the gate in that fence? Communication is *the* key. Do all you can to keep it as open as possible. Keep in mind that communication is only 8 percent verbal. The other 92 percent of communication is body language, eye contact, and tone of voice. You "speak" with 700,000 non-verbal ways. Your concern for your child is caught not taught.

Be honest from the start. That way, they will know they can trust your word later. Use the name of your HK's heart defect; it's floating all over the place. You may feel like that will frighten your child, but you can find the right words. Let children know that heart defects are serious, but it does not necessarily mean the person will die from it.

It Isn't Easy

It's not easy being the well one! Siblings need more than a quick "He's fine," so plan ahead what you'll tell them. They need information to help them understand what's going on. That's why communication isn't a one-time event. It's much more than just delivering the diagnosis. Keep sibs in the loop on their level. At times you might need to say something like this: "You probably noticed that John is really tired and grumpy lately. The medicines make him that way for right now. What do you think we could do to help him?"

Think about how important good information is to you. The adults in the family are usually processing information. Children need information to process also. Processing and talking through feelings is healthy for everyone. You may not realize how far down the road you have come, and without some information, children may be just beginning to deal with this new difficult journey.

Also, listen for misunderstandings. Explain procedures on the sib's level. Young children especially need to be reassured they did not cause the heart defect in any way — even if they've had "bad" thoughts and actions in the past against the HK. Also, let them know that heart defects are not contagious. Some adults may even think that ("Aren't *diseases* contagious?"). If needed, contact alternative support people (child life specialists, school counselors, teachers, chaplains, or church staff) for children to talk to. It may be easier to share feelings — especially negative ones — concerning the family, with a neutral third party. They may need to vent at times. Encourage your children to ask questions. Older children may even want to ask questions of the medical staff. Younger children may draw pictures, and then you can ask them to tell you about the picture. That is a great conversation starter.

In the hospital, three-year-old (HH) Caleb hadn't been able to see his baby brother. "They're hurting my baby. I want to see him." The nurse took a Polaroid picture of the mom, Allison, holding Nathan — swaddled, so Caleb couldn't see all the wires and scary things — except for the oxygen in his nose. Since the picture wasn't clear, he couldn't see things to upset him. Caleb carried around that picture for years.

Widening the Circle

Try to make sure the sibs don't miss school and their activities. Difficulties can arise with their friends because they can't relate to the heart defect experience. To make matters worse, you are less available to transport the siblings to visit friends or to other activities. Do what you can to facilitate their usual routines and activities. The usual people, places, and routines give "normalcy" to the day and provide a source of support and security for your children.

Communication is needed with teachers, coaches, and anyone who works with your child's siblings. *Forewarned is forearmed.* Talk with them to make sure they are aware of your family's situation. Or, if you need to have an assigned friend do this, let the teachers and others know that in writing, in an email, or by phone. Continue to keep teachers and coaches in the loop with e-mails or notes. Let them know what they can do to help. It's always better to take a proactive approach instead of just reacting to problems that arise.

Siblings' reaction to the heart defect stress may erupt in negative forms: anger, not doing work, pouting, withdrawing, and crying. All reactions depend on their individual personalities, and how things have been handled previously in their lives.

However, it's also possible for the siblings to demonstrate extreme positive behavior: stuffing negative feelings, overly conscientious, taking on extra responsibilities, and not wanting to add more burdens to the family. Let teachers and coaches know that you need to know from them what is happening with the siblings. They may say, "But you just have so much on you already." Express your appreciation, but explain that you can't help fix something if you don't know it's broken — that includes behavior and homework.

Because of extreme stress, a sibling may need help — and she probably wants one-on-one time with her parents. During certain stages with your heart child, you may not be able to give that time to the siblings. Include other adults in your children's lives and be appreciative of their involvement in your children's world. Just a brief note of thanks will make their day. These people play a crucial role and they're a positive piece of the puzzle. Let them know that.

Daily Routines

Routines create security for children, as their world has flipped upside down. Talk about regular routines; ask what they really miss that isn't happening now. You may be surprised how insignificant that routine may seem to you as an adult, but how important it is to the children. Review the "Love Languages" at the end of Resource One for clues as to why certain things are important to them.

The new normal includes a new routine, but it may be constantly changing. Explain any necessary changes that have to come into these new ravaged routines. Also, let the children know there may be changes that you can't let them know about beforehand, but you'll have a special time to talk with them afterwards. Transitions are especially difficult for introverted Blues (see Resource One),

"But we always read a story before bedtime," he may say. His very outgoing Yellow sibling probably won't care about transitions and changes as long as there are still people around to talk to.

Again, this is the new normal. Allow children to find ways to help and be included in the family's new routines. You can encourage the children by saying: "Things are not like they were before his heart defect — when things were normal. But we now have a new normal *and all of us will plan how we live it*. We're in this together." Try to be as positive as possible. They'll pick up on your attitude.

Acknowledge when their perceptions and thoughts are correct about what is happening in your HK's life and your family's life. They'll be able to trust their thoughts and ideas later in life as you reinforce them during this trying time. Many children feel that adults never listen to their ideas and opinions. Encourage your children to participate in the care of their heart sibling, both at home and in the hospital.

However, be careful not to put additional, unnecessary responsibility on the older ones or those who will say yes to whatever is asked. If possible, allow children to attend some clinic or hospital visits so that they can get to know the staff and receive some encouragement from them. Siblings can also spend time with their sister or brother in the hospital playing games, watching TV, and just spending quality time together.

Some may want to do that, and some may not. "He wants to act like nothing is going on. That's his way of coping," one mom said.

Emotional Landmines

Allow yourself to express your emotions in front of your children — to a certain point, depending on their ages and personalities. This delivers an important message: Mom gets frustrated and cries at times, so I can too. Catharsis, which is a feeling of release of an intense emotional experience, is important on this journey. Encourage your children to express their emotions openly and honestly with you. You both need a good catharsis.

However, the majority of the time you should let your children see a smile on your face — even if it is a forced smile. Still better, watch a funny movie together and laugh. Endorphins kick in and all of you need that.

Anger

There's a lot of potential for anger in the new normal. It may sound like this when it comes from your child's siblings:

* "Why can't my friends come over — they don't sneeze *that* much?"

* "Do I have to go with you to the doctor visit again with her (HK)?"

* "Why can't I just sleep in my own bed and have grandma come *here*?"

* "Grandma doesn't know the cereal I like or the PC games I play, and she can't help me with my math. She just sighs a lot."

* "My mom used to be nice. Now not so much."

What does anger sound like in *your* children? Keep your ears open for it. Here are some tips to help with your children's anger.

* Let children know it is okay to still have fun and do normal activities even though your family is coping with a CHD. Remember, laughter is healthy. It's hard to remember that at times, isn't it?

* Encourage your children to write in a journal or diary or draw pictures. This can provide a safe place for them to express their anger. (It can help them work through other negative emotions also.)

* Encourage physical activity. You will need to discuss how much or little your HK can do, and figure out ways to handle this subject with the siblings. Have the children (siblings) run laps around your yard, shoot baskets, or climb on a playground. They need to work through their feelings and concerns — not bottle them up. You do too, by the way.

＊ Maintain consistent discipline with all of your children (no matter what the negative reactions are). Boundaries give the stability and security they all need.

Jealousy

Siblings may think, "He gets everything, even mom." Then the guilt kicks in and the next thought may be, "How could I think that?"

One sibling said, "How do you live up to 'the legend' who has so much courage? I can never be what he is."

Jealousy may look like this: Your HK has been throwing up for hours and then your well one throws up a little. Your HK is fatigued, and then your well one is tired all the time and wants to cuddle. It's past midnight and your HK is wired on meds, you pop in a DVD to pass the time, and guess who shows up at the bedroom door? "I just can't sleep," the well one mumbles.

"But those actions are psychosomatic. They're not real," one mom said.

The truth is that they are very real to the sufferer. If you encounter a situation like that, do whatever it takes to spend time with the sib. Say, "I'm so sorry you don't feel well. Let's wrap you in this quilt and snuggle. What would taste good to you?" The cure for jealousy is time and attention. Even small doses help.

Frustration

We asked many siblings what advice or tips they would give to other siblings. The answer?

"One word: Patience! Know that you aren't in the spotlight, at all. That your parents are doing the best they can, and are probably worried about finances, jobs, and having to deal with a child with a heart defect. Just have patience."

"People grab your arm at church, school, everywhere and say, 'How is he doing?' I don't really like to have my arm grabbed all the time, but I've learned to just smile, give them a short, planned answer and say, 'Thank you for asking.'"

Another sib said, "Everyone says, 'How are you doing?' I feel like saying, 'Lousy! How are you doing?' Actually, that isn't totally true. The people who've gone through this say other things. I can't remember what they are; just that it doesn't make me mad."

Talking to a child life specialist or counselor may also alleviate a child's concerns or frustrations. Again, it may help him cope and carve out his own identity — not just "John's brother."

Loneliness

An older sibling may spend many hours home alone. She may be microwaving meals by herself. If grandma and friends come in it helps, but not always. The older sibling may be torn between "I don't need a babysitter" and feeling like nothing can replace the family that is usually there. Take time to talk to these "almost adults" about their feelings.

Keep the siblings (whatever age) with you as a family as much as possible. Sharing Jell-O on a hospital tray beats anything, anywhere, at times. Reassure your children that they will be cared for no matter what happens. You may feel that they surely know that. But they don't. A heart defect has thrown everything into upheaval, and, mainly, they just want you — no matter what their age.

Fear

The underlying emotion in most siblings is fear. Fear of HK's condition and death; fear that parents may get sick and die, too; fear that they will be left alone. Assure them (repeatedly) that someone will always be there to take care of them.

Filling the Tanks

Show your children that you love them by filling those tanks again — and again and again. What are their love languages? (Review the end of Resource One.) Here are some ways to show your love and fill those emotional tanks:

* Touch. This includes hugs for teens too.

* Time. Stop, look (eye to eye), and listen. Don't just mumble, "Uh huh." Ask where the sib would like to spend time with you.

✶ Talk. Encouraging words give courage to keep on keeping on. They may get daily doses of discouraging words in life. "I love you, honey" written on a sticky note, and tucked inside a math book can make a huge difference to a hurting t'ween.

✶ Gifts. Not particularly expensive. Just something to say, "I'm thinking about you." Choose something meaningful just for them.

✶ Deeds. What do the children do? Thank them for those acts, and find things to do for them. When we asked sibs, "What was a big help to your family?" many said the same thing. "People brought food!" Deeds done in love. We all need to receive those.

Two more helpful books by Gary Chapman are *Five Love Languages of Children* and *Five Love Languages of Teenagers*. They make good reading in the middle of the night.

Dear Reader, as you hold this book in your hands, rest assured you have been prayed for by the author and fellow travelers. You and your family are important to us. We pray that these words encourage you as you affect the lives of your children — HKs and well ones. We pray that He will sweep away the fog, give you clarity to view each child, and strength to meet those needs — one step at a time. Again, you are precious to us and more so to Him. He is the one who gives us others who come alongside.

...and the peace of God, which surpasses all understanding,
will guard your hearts and minds through Christ Jesus.
Philippians 4:7

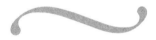

Blessed are they who have the gift of making friends,
for it is one of God's best gifts. It involves many things,
but above all, the power of going out of one's self, and appreciate
whatever is noble and loving in another.

— Helen Keller

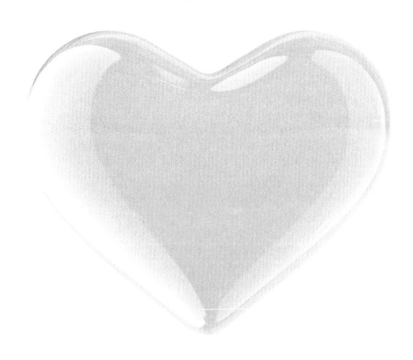

Chapter Ten

Friends: The Family You Choose

Like an elastic bandage wrapped snuggly around a sprained ankle, giving support during the healing process, so friends wrap around you and provide support during your healing process as you deal with your child's journey. Friends don't squeeze too tight and smother you, but they do give you strength as you continue to function. Allow them that privilege. Don't let them miss the blessing.

Strength and Support

Friends are "family," not by blood or marriage, but by love. Sometimes they're closer than relatives in location and in relationships. They help you carry the burden and get the job done. Like the support that family offers, friends do the same. They bring so many positives into a difficult situation. Many parents noted that friends

111

bring food, pick up the kids, transport the siblings to and from extracurricular activities, and take them out for fun. They bring groceries and put them away, lug in cleaning supplies to scrub toilets, and throw in a load of wash. Friends also provide spiritual support and prayer.

One mom said, "No matter how bad things have gotten, just being with these church 'sisters' helps me remember that this world isn't the end."

Another said, "I have to set limits on how long I unload on some friends. I can completely drain them without realizing it."

Then there are those friends who visit at inconvenient times...for them. You know they've left family at home, left work undone, but choose to be with you — and you are thankful to have them at your side.

Stay a While, My Friend

Stay a while my friend
Just sit and talk.
I don't care about what — just talk.
Tell me about your outside world
I know it still exits.

Just stay a while
Sit and listen.
Listen to my fears, my dark thoughts
The ones that strike late afternoon.
The shifts change, the day people leave
The night people scurry down the hall
Checking charts, shoving stacked carts
So much to do, so much to do....

So, stay a while
The dark comes soon
And if I talk and listen to you
I can make it till the night.
Then curl up on the sleep/sofa
Doze as the flickering TV light fades.
Susan's IV alarm beeps and buzzes soon enough
I'll hit the buttons — she'll wake and whimper
Two hours sleep last night.
So for now
Please stay a while, my friend.

Root Wrapping

Majestic redwoods grow in groups of five and their shallow roots intertwine. This enables trees to survive severe storms that blow in from the Pacific. Like redwoods, heart families root wrap, enabling them to survive severe storms. Root wrapping starts in waiting rooms — continues in hospital halls, support groups, chat rooms, e-mails, and phone calls.

"I hate to say to the new parents on the floor, 'Welcome to the club that none of us wanted to join,'" said a mom. "It's a bizarre world with a secret language."

Here's what some parents say about the club that no one wanted to join:

* There's no president, it's all equal opportunity, no matter what you have or don't have. Some families are wealthy; some have absolutely nothing of this world's goods. But all families feel the same helplessness when they hear the diagnosis.

* There's no secretary, but you need to keep your own daily journal including meds, reactions to the meds, and helpful hints for hospital staff caring for your child. You are your child's best advocate.

* There's no treasurer, all the money is out-go, not income — except from generous friends and organiza-tions. Ask the social workers and other pro-fessionals at the hospi-tal to help you locate organizations and help if needed.

Helps & Hope

God's Promise

*Let each of you look out
not only for his own interests,
but also for the interests of others.*
— Philippians 2:4

* No one ever looks forward to welcoming new members; we hope our club will become extinct. Once you're admitted, you have a lifetime membership in the club. The upside of that is you have others who really understand and encourage you (which helps you endure being in the club).

Some of you have just joined this club, others have been members a short while, and others for as long as you can remember.

Whatever length of time, please take advantage of others in the club. They're there for you — night and day.

"It's amazing how giving brings such huge returns. We don't do it for that, but it just works that way. Welcome to the club."

It Was the Best of Times; It Was the Worst of Times....

There are no mind readers. Let them know how you are feeling — that there will be times you want to talk, and times you really don't. There will be times you want those close friends to get messag-es to others, and times you want them to keep it to them-selves. There will be times

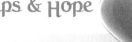

Helps & Hope

God's Promise

*Praise be to... the God of all
comfort, who comforts us in all our
troubles, so that we can comfort
those in any trouble with the
comfort we ourselves have received
from God.*
— 2 Corinthians 1:3-4

you want to hear about their "normal" lives, and times you don't. There will be times you want to hear about their problems, and times you had rather not. Only you can tell someone what you need at that time. One mom suggested pinning on the appropriate button, "Thanks, but I don't want to talk now," or "Please let me talk and cry — but just listen."

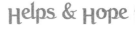

Kindred Spirits — Lifeline Connections
(Joanie and Gregg, Glenna and Tom — their story)

Joanie: "We were introduced to Glenna and Tom by the pastor at the church we started attending right after we found out our baby girl had a serious heart defect. We had lots in common with vocations — teaching, athletics, coaching, and the main thing we shared was being parents of a heart child, but we still had our baby. Their son had died three years before that.

"I couldn't believe when Glenna and Tom came to visit us in the children's hospital — the very hospital where their baby boy had passed away. I knew she hadn't gone back there since that time, and I was concerned for all the memories that would hit. But they came, and have been steadfast friends ever since."

Glenna: "We wanted God to use something so painful in our lives, and I needed something good to come out of being in the same children's hospital, and same doctors — so we needed *to be there* for Joanie and Gregg and their family. We've shared ups, downs, ins, and outs with them for over twenty years."

Gregg: "I sat with Tom and asked him, 'What do you do if *it* happens?'"

Gregg knew Tom had survived the death of his son, and he was standing by Gregg in his child's heart journey. They'd played sports, coached, and prayed together, and now shared the heart journey.

Men, if you have been on this journey for a while, look for the new dads who are reeling — trying to be strong for their families. Many times it is more difficult for men to open up to others — but you take the first step and offer that special gift of friendship — from one who has been there.

"Tom has been there for us — and his walk with the Lord has given me strength for our journey. He lives what he says."

More Kindred Spirits

"Nurse Nancy brought our four families together," Colleen said.

In November and December of 2000, four baby boys were born with a very rare and serious heart defect called Hypoplastic Left Heart Syndrome (HLHS) — and all four families lived within fifteen miles of each other. None of these families knew the others or knew much about CHDs. All four underwent their first open-heart surgery, the Norwood procedure (part of a three-part surgical repair required to re-route their tiny hearts), and then were sent home. They were followed by the same home care nurse, Nancy — who helped ease the minds of parents and made sense of confusing medication schedules. After their surgeries and recoveries, she began checking on these little boys and commented on the four boys, all with HLHS, and they lived so close to one another. Telephone numbers were asked for and connections to last-a-lifetime began.

"We've shared laughter, tears, dinners, birthdays, heart walks, parties, hospital visits, but most of all friendship and support," Colleen continued. "Unfortunately, we've also shared deep sorrows as we attended the funeral of one of four little heart friends, seven-year-old Evan. The service was unbelievably moving, incredibly sad, and yet so comforting all at once. The pastor said, 'From the day they are born and placed in our arms, we should immediately give them back into God's hands and pray that His will be done. And, thank Him for giving you the privilege of being their earthly parent for whatever length of time He gives you.'

"As time went on we welcomed other heart families into our group, and we are now, Hearts of Hope, www.heartsofhopemi.org. We are friends from the heart, and Nurse Nancy is 'our angel'."

Take a few moments to think about the "coincidences" God has brought into your life on this journey. Who are the friends you're root wrapping with — and what have they done for you? What have you had the opportunity to do for them? Who are the kindred spirits you've made on your heart journey? Thank Him for His "coincidences" — and for all the others God will bring into your life and your child's life in the future. Now meet more new friends in the new place.

You shall love your neighbor as yourself.
Galatians 5:14

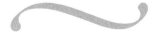

Alone we can do so little; together we can do so much.

— Helen Keller

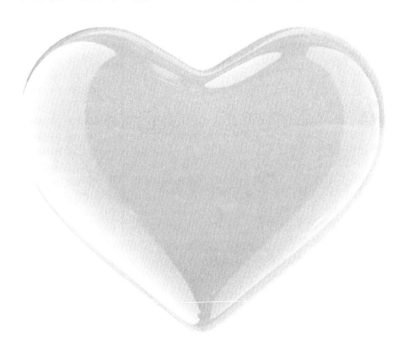

Chapter Eleven

Hospital Hospital-ity

Hospitals, especially children's hospitals have changed greatly over the years — but key ingredients remain — caring and healing. Healing is dispensed, not only in the pharmacy, but also through the staff as they meet needs: physical, emotional, and spiritual. How do you react to the staff and *their* needs?

Back to the Future

* In 1944, the first "blue baby" operation launched a golden age of heart surgery. As they operated and new blood began to flow into the infant's heart, they took off the sheets and saw the child's color change from blue to pink. "It's a miracle," someone said. The film *Something the Lord*

Made documents the development of the first operative procedure on a congenital heart abnormality. It opened the door to heart surgery for the future.

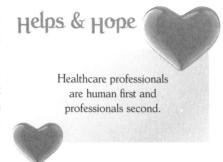

Helps & Hope

Healthcare professionals are human first and professionals second.

✳ In 1959, nurses in Ohio spent a sleepless night, despite their months of practice. Most went to the chapel in the morning to pray — aware of what was in their hands — a child's life. It was a new feeling. They were walking into uncertain waters, one mistake could cost a child her life, and they were scared to death. They assisted in Dayton's first open heart surgery — a seven hour operation — requiring six doctors, six nurses, and three technicians — all to repair a hole in a nine-year-old girl's heart.

Today's Team

"My child is so sick, how can I think of anyone else?"

Overwhelmed parents may have little patience in dealing with the humanness of hospital staffs. However, hospital staffs are human. They have their own families, health issues, and stress factors — not the least of which is working in a children's hospital. As you interact with these new people in the new place, review Resource One on personalities, which will help you understand them better as individuals. Remember that you're all on the same team, working toward the same goal — to help your child.

You know how frustrated you feel when you ask the doctors your 'why' questions and they reply, "We don't really know why." On the other side of that fence, they too want to know the answer to the whys, and they devote their lives to finding those answers. They deal with the whys every day. Your pain is their pain too.

Around tables at staff meetings and grabbing one-on-one sessions in the hall, these professionals wrestle with difficult questions and plans-of-action in a field where there are few guideposts and fewer guarantees. Some smile, give hugs, and shed tears with you;

others appear reserved and only give objective answers. Some days your smile may not be returned, but keep giving it away. You never know what is happening in someone else's life.

In 2005, after hurricane Katrina devastated the gulf coast, the New Orleans Children's Hospital posted this page on their website. It spoke volumes.

"Everyone continues to put all of the personal loss behind them and tend to the patients, our first priority. It is only in the silence of a broken heart, when alone for a few minutes, or with a trusted co-worker, that the tears flow briefly, and then it is back to business. I do believe that most of the patients do not know the extent of the loss of the healthcare workers that are caring for them. And, they shouldn't know it. It should not be their burden."

A Hospital Tour

Welcome to a children's hospital: kid-sized and child friendly. As you enter the doors, you're bombarded by vibrant colors splashed across the walls, ceiling, floors, doors, and chairs. Red wagons and wheelchairs, along with IV poles and pumps, are maneuvered through the mazelike halls by parents, siblings, volunteers, and staff. Each hospital is unique, but the same in the most important way. They all state, "We're here for each child."

As you meet the staff along the way, give them a huge gift — a smile! This is especially needed if they're not wearing one. They may not have seen one in a long time, as each of their days is stitched with concern for all the children in their care. Another huge gift to give staff is to pray for them each day. Pray for wisdom as they make decisions affecting the children in their care, and pray for them and their families. God knows their individual needs. Who are the people on the staff? Keep your eyes open.

Parking Garage

The mom drove into the hospital's parking garage, came to a stop, and pushed the familiar ticket button. She pulled the ticket from the machine, the yellow-striped security arm rose, and she began the ascent. Level 1A, slowly circling; 1B, no spots; 2A, circle; 2B, not anything yet; 3A, 3B, someone pulling out?; 4A, 4B, 5A, 5B, 6A, last chance before the off-limits helicopter pad; 6A, an open spot!

Mom unharnessed her sleeping child from the car seat, lifted his slumping weight, and shifted him on to her shoulder. Then she grabbed the diaper bag (which served as a carryall) and threw it over her other shoulder, balancing herself out. She trudged to the elevator, pushed the button, and waited — and waited. Thus began another day dealing with a gamut of people and procedures. Today she was headed toward the clinic — where waiting had become an art form.

Information Desk

Stepping out of the elevator, many families need assistance with directions. Help usually is nearby — information and a smile — delivered from the information desk.

One person who worked the information desk said, "People wander off the elevators with that lost look. They think they should know answers to simple questions, but many don't. Everything is scary and new, but it's old to us. Their minds are crowded with concerns for their child, and they just need a friendly face to let them know we're here to help. I'm blessed to come alongside these people each day.

One day a mommy just stood there and cried, and as we talked, no phones rang! That had to be God working. My husband said I have a Kleenex ministry."

These people answer questions and attempt to listen — between umpteen phone calls.

One staffer said, "If we can alleviate any of their trauma, then we've done our job. And we want them to know that as long as there's life, there's hope."

Chaplains

According to the dictionary, a chaplain is a member of the clergy employed to give religious guidance, but they do much more than that. One of their more important roles is to offer a kind, listening, ear.

"We had no choice in this horrendous journey, but they [chaplains] choose to enter our pain," a mom said.

"And we are privileged to do so," the chaplain responded.

Chaplains are usually the first line of spiritual help in the hospital, ministering to patients, parents, and staff.

Chaplains minister to groups and to individual families as they serve in the trenches everyday.

Doctors

"I don't know how these doctors (and staff) do this job. I can't imagine choosing to deal with childhood heart defects day in and day out," a mom said.

"I don't know how these parents deal with this day in and day out," a staff person replied.

Both appreciate the horrendous task each carries. Both put the child's welfare above their own. Both encourage the other's role in this part of the journey, thereby giving courage to persevere.

One mom said, "When you've hit the wall — again — don't see your doctor as the enemy. Appreciate the responsibilities that he has; he determines the whole course of treatment for your child. Decisions are made by the team, but this person's opinion will shape everything."

Doctor's schedules are packed, so do your homework, keeping up on new information on the Internet (but be selective of the sites — ask a professional for their suggestions.) If you come across more helpful information, ask for a consultation with the doctor. Don't grab the doctor in the hall or when they're making rounds if you need to discuss your child's situation more in depth. Value their time and expertise. You're on the same team.

One mom said, "I told our doctor, 'You have my most prized possession (my daughter) in the world.' He said he kept remembering my words. He was our advocate from day one."

How do you relate to the doctors taking care of your child?

Some parents say, "She's the doctor, the professional. I'm just the mom."

Keep in mind that you're a team. Your child needs an advocate (you) to keep watch on her meds, feelings (you know her better than anyone), and all the day-by-day issues. Healthcare professionals are human. Many times they are overworked and weary.

Occasionally mistakes happen — not on purpose. So you can

help them by keeping track in a journal of medications, reactions to those medications, and methods to use. This protects and benefits your child, the staff, and you.

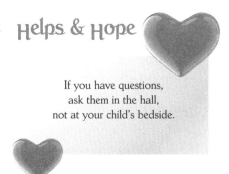

Other parents express a sentiment like this one: "I've never trusted doctors, and you better believe I'm double-checking everything going on. My baby (age seventeen) had a bad reaction to that new medication they gave him. Seems like they'd know better."

All it takes is one outburst or negative comment to undermine your child's confidence in his medical care. You want the best healing situation for him, not the worst.

And no matter how stressed you are, remember you're addressing a fellow human being who cares about your child — one who is on his care team.

Nurses

Nurses serve on the front line of the battle and few understand the thoughts, feelings, and fears of the patients and families better than they. Each patient's journey is unique in changes and challenges. Every day brings new twists in the road.

One nurse, Mary Ann, tells her story, recounting her days as a pediatric oncology nurse. "I just couldn't understand it. People said, 'We really depend on you as our nurse and appreciate all you do for us.' I loved their children, and this was my job. I just never expected that love to be returned. I always felt that I was the lucky one to have come in contact with these families."

Mary Ann left nursing as her family expanded, and they moved to another state. Then baby number six was born — with a severe heart defect.

"They gave this precious child two years to live," Mary Ann said. "Our world fell apart, and I began to experience life from the other side (as the parent of a critically ill child). On the first night of Megan's diagnosis, I was still reeling from what the doctor had told me — and totally unprepared for what I knew (from a nurse's perspective) would be happening to my baby. We walked into the intensive care unit and the nurses called Megan by her first name. That simple act was so important to me. I'm not sure if I could have left her with them if she had just been a number. For some reason, it made me feel as if they cared and would really treat her that way — and they never let me down. As the nurses came and went out of our room 24/7, I finally understood what the parents years ago were telling me. I depended on the nurses and appreciated each small kindness shown to us. It was often the nurses who picked up the pieces when I was left in tears after listening to the doctor and the situation with our child. Being the recipient gave me a whole new appreciation for being a nurse, and I'll never forget the nurses who cared for our child." Mary Ann has experienced both sides, helping and being helped.

Recognize and appreciate the balance you experience in nurses' personalities. Some are laid back, and others are hyper-vigilant, alert and looking for problems that might arise. Each has their own strengths in personality and giftedness. Express your gratitude for them individually — they are there to help you and your child.

"The nurses thought of everything," Allison (a mom) said. "I was so lucky to get to nurse my baby when he was in the NICU. Many heart babies can't nurse because they don't have the strength to do so. I was led down the hall to a special room that was a pumping station — all fitted with a comfortable recliner, sterilized kits, and a refrigerator filled with juices and water bottles to keep me hydrated."

"We need to take care of you, so we can take care of your baby. Drink up," a nurse said.

"I felt so out of control on our new journey, and to experience all the help the staff gave, filled me with relief and confidence that I needed so desperately."

Intensa Care Nurse
We didn't know when we left Georgia in 1985 to go to another state for our six-year-old son Matt's second surgery that we

wouldn't come home with him. The first surgery there had gone well, and he'd lived a normal life, even with his rare heart defect. This was a total shock. When I think of that hospitalization, one kindness stands out in the fog we endured — it was a special ICU nurse named Miss Jackie.

Matt had a very rare heart defect, and she had taken care of him for his first surgery and touched his life in the ICU with her comfort and kindness. She bought him an autograph dog and had the staff to sign it. When we arrived for the second surgery, Matt asked his surgeon if he could have Miss Jackie as his nurse. (We found out she wasn't on that unit anymore.)

"Let me see what I can do, bud," was his answer.

Then to make sure she would come, Matt handwrote a note on a Wendy's® napkin,

"Miss Jackie. Will you be my intensa care nurse? Matt."

Miss Jackie got the word — and the napkin request. She was by his side the last day of his life here on earth. Not only did she touch his life, and us — his parents, but also our eleven-year-old daughter Jennifer, as she said, "I saw the comfort she gave to my brother, and I wanted to be a nurse." And today, she's a nurse who gives comfort to her patients.

Phlebotomist

"It was our first night in the hospital and I asked the phlebotomist why they had to take Nathan's blood at 4am," Allison (mom) said. "She told me they had to get the results ready for the doctors who came later on rounds. She was only on the floor for thirty minutes, so I asked if there was any way she could make those 'sticks' easier. She said she'd stop by his room when she first came on the floor and put the EMLA cream where she'd take the stick. The cream deadened the pain- and she put a patch over it so he wouldn't rub it off. She then came back at the end of the time and took the blood. Well, time she got back, Nathan was sound asleep, she took the blood, and he didn't feel a thing — he slept right through it. I really appreciated her changing things around. She really wanted to help these children however she could."

Social Worker

One of the computer support staff at the hospital said, "A friend talked me into walking up a small local mountain. Being a veteran climber, she set a pace that I struggled, breathless, to follow. As the summit came into sight, I stopped to massage my cramping legs and suck in some much needed air. I told her I couldn't finish the hike. She didn't respond the way many people would, by saying, 'Sure you can.' Instead she simply said, 'Give me your hand.' I gladly accepted her help and her strength, and we finished the climb hand in hand."

Helps & Hope

Social workers also assist with resources, advocacy, financial issues, family interactions, and problem solving.

Social workers are there to give you a hand, especially when you've reached your limit. When your cramping legs, shortness of breath, and despairing thoughts scream, "Just give up," these professionals extend a hand. They will help you on this journey inside the hospital and outside as you go home. They've been trained to do this. They have climbed this mountain with others, and they are there to give you strength and guidance on this difficult climb. Grab their hand.

Child Life Specialist

"We're basically 'distracters' who bring toys and sometimes sing to the child during procedures and doctor's appointments," a child life specialist said. "We help the child and family to learn positive coping skills, and reduce anxiety while going through treatment."

Play, art, music therapy, and puppets help children understand their illness and medical procedures. They can express their feelings and simply have fun. "We're also there to help celebrate important events in the child's life, such as birthdays and accomplishing goals set by families and staff."

Outside of their hospital rooms, playrooms and TeenZones are safe, supportive places where patients and siblings can enjoy special activities and entertainment. No medical procedures are allowed in rooms identified as "safe places."

Healthy children experience play as a normal part of life. For ill children, play is even more important; it helps them cope with their overwhelming experiences in the hospital.

The "ists" and "gists"

There are many "ists" — some are therapists, nutritionists, pharmacists — and there are many "gists" — such as cardiologists and radiologists. They all play crucial roles in your child's life. Thank the "ists" and the "gists" as they interact with you and your child.

Volunteers

"You've got quite a load in that wagon," a man on the elevator said. The volunteer was delivering a mound of new toys to the children on the third floor.

"You can't give without receiving," she said.

Volunteers give of their time and help with hundreds of tasks to come alongside the hospital staff.

"We'd never be able to do all the things we do without the hundreds of volunteers," the volunteer coordinator said. "They give us extra sets of hands and listening ears, and they give love to the children and their parents. They enjoy bringing smiles to the children's faces — especially to those who seldom smile.

"Some parents and older siblings of HKs and even the HKs themselves want to come back to the hospital to volunteer once their stay is over. They really want to give back," the coordinator explained.

A volunteer who was a retired nurse said, "Things are so different in children's hospitals today. I watched a little boy with a small remote-controlled car weaving serpentine down the hall. The staff gingerly stepped over the car and never complained. I couldn't believe it. Years ago, someone would have grabbed him up and taken him to his room. It's amazing how the staff works around and with the patients."

Educational support

Some children's hospitals have classrooms, schoolteachers, and volunteers. They give normalcy for about three hours, five days a week. The HK feels as if there is a future beyond heart defects as he accomplishes tasks, and it pays off later when he returns to school. He's not far behind in his work; maybe he'll even be caught up — whether he attends public/private school or is homeschooled.

What if the HK just doesn't feel like coming to school? Bedside tutoring can bring school to them. This gives parents and other caregivers a break to leave the room while the schoolroom tutor works with the child.

However, a teacher in one children's hospital says, "Bedside instruction isn't for the one who just doesn't feel like coming to the classroom. The medical staff must say he/she can't come — that they are too sick, (which usually means too sick for anything) can't leave the room because of medication which needs constant monitoring and other issues."

Often, individual instruction helps the shy/easily overwhelmed kid with new concepts and skills, as well as, remediates, and fills in gaps caused by (school) absences and illness.

Overwhelmed parents may not think schoolwork is important; there are too many other issues demanding their attention. but, this is something parents and HKs can assert some control over, and controlling anything on this journey is worth the effort.

More Initials

NICU- Neonatal Intensive Care Unit
CICU- Cardiac Intensive Care Unit
PICU- Pediatric Intensive Care Unit

Children in intensive care units are monitored, checked on, and given constant care by the medical staff. They are loved on, prayed over, tucked in, and sung to by parents and other loved ones. Everyone could use some "intensive" care in their lives, but these children need it more so.

Environmental Services

Those who come to clean the rooms are on the journey too. They observe the extreme pain in lives of children and parents every day as they do their jobs.

One grandfather brightened a custodial staff member's day when he said, "I can't imagine what this room would look like if you didn't do your job!"

Cafeteria

"I need one hand to pull the wagon, and one to steer the IV pole, and one to push my tray. I've run out of hands," the dad said in the cafeteria line. If possible, plan ahead for trips to the cafeteria and places requiring more than two hands to maneuver. Give those who work there a smile over the steam table, or as you hand them money in the check-out line.

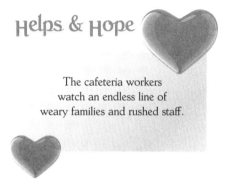

Helps & Hope

The cafeteria workers watch an endless line of weary families and rushed staff.

Family Resource Center

Whether you're looking for research on your child's disease, a novel for yourself, children's books, videos and DVDs, or a computer to use, these are the people to ask and this is the place to come.

Gift Shop

Necessities, magazines, books, toys, and cards can all be found here. It's probably the only store within walking distance. Take advantage — it may be your only "outing" for weeks at a time.

When you began this journey you didn't know your way around the hospital. Where is the cafeteria? Where is the family resource center? Where is the gift shop? With time, you're passing this information on to others who ask the same questions. In fact, you've joined a new family — the hospital family. Courage increases for each one on this journey as encouragement passes from member to member.

For we walk by faith, not by sight...
2 Corinthians 5:7

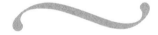

*You alone can do your grief work,
but you do not have to do it alone.*

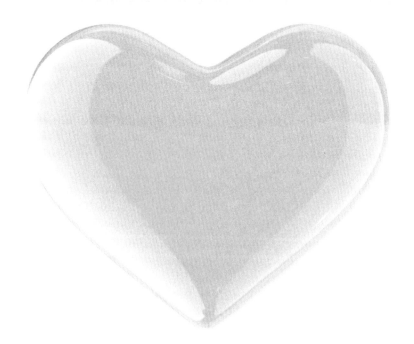

Chapter Twelve

You're Not Alone

L isa's Story (Part One)

If you are reading this book, then you are, more than likely, a fellow traveler on the journey. If your CDH child has died, as mine has, then I can only tell you, I am so very sorry for your loss. I've been where you are.

What you are going through now is harder than anything you'll ever experience again in your life. You may feel that you can't survive it. But you will. You may feel that you don't *want* to survive it. Those feelings will pass — even if you don't believe that right now — in this moment. Nothing that I, or any other fellow traveler, can tell you will make it all better, but we can walk the journey with you, and help you to understand where you are on the road. How do we do that? Only by sharing our own experiences on the same journey.

In February of 1983, our youngest daughter, Elizabeth Anne — our Betsie--was born six weeks early, with Transposition of the Great Vessels/Total Anomalous Pulmonary Venous Return. Big words that meant nothing to me, except that her heart was all wrong.

Within twelve hours of her birth she'd been rushed to the University of Texas Health Science Center at San Antonio for balloon septostomy to enlarge the tiny opening between the ventricles so that she could receive more oxygenated blood. We were told this was a stop-gap procedure to *save her life*, and buy us some time, but that there would be many, many more *surgeries* to come, *if she survived*.

I remember gazing at her in the isolette and marveling at how tiny she was in comparison to her three-year-old sister and 18 month old brother, and yet, at four pounds, 15 ounces, she looked like an elephant baby compared to the teeny-tiny preemies in the NICU. And she was a Xerox copy of her big sister. Shrunk down to miniature, but a little clone — such a sweet face.

The next seven days are a jumble of memories — little sleep, no food that I can recall, pumping my breasts so they could tube feed the baby, because she would "burn too many calories if we let her suck."

On the sixth day, my husband, Richard, encouraged me to stay home — rest awhile. She was holding her own, so I did. That's when the call came.

"Mrs. Hauser, Elizabeth is in congestive heart failure. We're trying to bring her out of it with meds, but we need to make some decisions."

The decision they wanted us to make was to do open-heart surgery to repair the baby's heart the next day — not a year down the road when she had grown enough to survive the surgery — that's what we'd been aiming for.

"She will continue to go into CHF. Every time it happens it damages the heart muscle more. We can, *more than likely*, bring her out if it with meds, but by the time we think she's big enough, there may not be enough healthy heart left, on which to operate. We need to do this now."

I signed the consent form. Me. I did it. Myself. With my own hand.

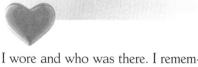

Helps & Hope

There are no words that make you feel better when your child has died. *I'm so sorry,* comes the closest.

Elizabeth Anne Hauser, aged 8 days, daughter of Richard and Lisa Kay Hauser, did not survive the surgery. Her heart stopped and my life shattered.

I don't remember the funeral service. I remember what I wore and who was there. I remember walking from the car to the graveside, then nothing until we were half-way back across the parking lot to the car, but nothing about the service. I'm still sad about that.

I remember the crush of family and friends who rallied around us. How they tried to help, and couldn't. How they offered well-intentioned, but inadequate words. Not because they weren't trying, but because there are no words.

What I remember the most is being angry: angry at the doctors because they didn't fix her; angry at Richard because he wasn't grieving like I was, angry at myself because I signed those stupid papers — I was the mommy and should have been able to kiss her and make her better; and angry at God because He had allowed it to happen in the first place. I couldn't do anything about the doctors or God, but I sure could take it out on Richard!

And I did. The colder and more distant he became, the harder and louder I cried. It was as though he wasn't going to grieve — so I had to do it for both of us. He wasn't going to talk about Betsie, so I talked about her and her short life non-stop. It must have tortured him. I know it tortured me.

I ran the pregnancy through my mind over and over again. What could I have done differently? Eaten better? Slept more? Less caffeine? More milk? The woulda, coulda, shoulda's will eat you alive.

One day Richard snapped, "Lisa, when are you going to get over this?"

"I don't know! I've never had a dead baby before!" I screeched.

Because Betsie was six weeks premature, we hadn't even arrived at her due date yet. I still had milk in my breasts. I was a raging pack of hormones and grief and post-partum depression. Not pretty.

Someone suggested Compassionate Friends. This group is made up of bereaved parents by bereaved parents for bereaved parents. We went to our first meeting. There were two

other new couples there for the first time that night. One of the other fathers was quite vocal and shared a lot about what he was feeling. Richard is not a big "sharer," but I think that dad's openness touched Richard. When someone asked how he was handling things, he swallowed hard, then leaned forward in his chair and looked at his shoes.

"I get really ticked off when people ask me, 'How's Lisa doing' like I didn't lose the baby, too."

All my anger at my husband melted away in that moment.

I'm so very thankful for Compassionate Friends. I think they probably saved my marriage.

No matter where you are on your journey — whether you are in the dark, dark early days, or beginning to move toward more lighter days — I hope you'll connect with other parents who have walked this journey before you.

As you make your way, in these early days, you'll find comfort in some of God's smallest blessings. I can't promise that "time heals all wounds," but as it goes by, it does offer perspective. You will never "get over" losing your precious child, but I promise that there will come a day when you'll be able to laugh out loud again, without guilt.

Remember that there are others who have walked this road before you, and who are willing to walk it with you now. Seek us out. We care, and we want you to know that **You are not alone!**

Grief is Loss

"Grief is loss no matter what you've lost," Martha said. "We went through the 'grief steps' from the first heart diagnosis, and many times since then. We've watched other heart families work through the steps on their journey, and some with the final loss of their child here on earth."

Life on planet earth is a journey. Somehow, we think that journey should always be smooth. We'll accept a few bumps, but we certainly don't expect to be plunged into fearful tunnels. When that happens, we reel in the darkness and want answers — and solutions. Others want to give us those answers and help us see solutions. However, many times the answers don't come quickly, but the waiting can pull us to Him.

In April 1995, a jarring blast rocked Oklahoma City — the bombing of the Murrah Federal Building. Nearby, the First United Methodist Church suffered massive destruction, including its elaborate stained-glass windows. Now restored, one of the windows in the church's chapel was created from shards of stained glass. Worked into the breathtaking new window are these words. "The Lord takes broken pieces and by His love makes us whole."

Listen to Paul's words in 2 Corinthians 4:8-9. He had an advanced degree in suffering:

We are hard-pressed on every side, yet not crushed; we are perplexed, but not in despair; persecuted; but not forsaken; struck down, but not destroyed —

Stages of Grief

These stages are a reminder that others have walked this road before you. Be alert though. Stages may not come in a neat order, and stages that you've already walked through may hit again — unexpectedly.

(Taken from *Chronic Kids, Constant Hope.*)

✳ During **Denial and Isolation**:

Recite your child's diagnosis over and over. Write it down. Call a friend and repeat it.

Why? You'll stay somewhat "stuck" in this stage and find it difficult to move through the other stages if you haven't yet accepted the reality of the condition.

✴ During **Anger**:

Do something physically creative or safely aggressive — finger-paint in bright colors, punch pillows, pound the piano. Go into the woods and scream — or split some logs.

✴ During **Bargaining**:

Write out a promise to yourself and the Lord — something you can and will do regardless of the outcome of your child's diagnosis. It might be memorizing a specific verse or rereading a chapter in a favorite comforting book.

✴ During **Depression**:

A feeling of numbness, anger, and sadness may lurk underneath. Buy yourself fresh flowers (have a jar of change collecting specifically for these times). Go to a bookstore and give yourself an hour to browse. Find a creative project small enough to complete in a short time (even baking bread) to give yourself a feeling of accomplishment. Eat chocolate! (That comes with a warning, however.)

✴ During **Acceptance**:

Record your feelings and emotions in your journal. Mark the date on your calendar. Return to the journal entry when you find yourself retracing the steps of grief.

And of course, you need to be aware of your other children, the siblings walking alongside you through the grief process. Although you're grieving, they still need your presence and comfort. Furthermore, they may not experience the stages of grief in the order that you do. Allow them to grieve in their own way.

Someone said, "You alone can do your grief work, but you do not have to do it alone."

God Himself comes alongside us to help, and He sends fellow travelers to do the same. They offer shining rays of hope — sometimes in unexpected ways.

Lisa's Story (Part Two)

In those first dark hours after Betsie died, it seemed almost as if time stood still. It was a mish-mash of decisions and activities; of phone calls and preparations; the visit to the funeral home; then picking up our other two toddlers; of friends and family coming in and out of our little house. And the tears — so many tears. I see all of that

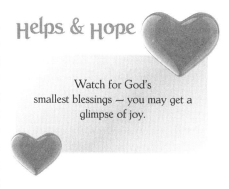

as though through a mist. There is only one thing that stands out distinctly in my memory: the call from my grandmother.

My grandmother was my touchstone. She was the most grace-filled woman I've ever known. I strive to be like her because she was so special. In a span of a year and a half, she lost her husband, a four-year-old son, and her beloved mother-in-law. Yet, she held onto her faith, and her joy for life. Several years later, she married my granddad and their first baby was born with a congenital heart defect. He died three hours after his birth.

When the phone rang that day in my kitchen, I didn't want to talk to one more person. But it was my grandmother. "Honey," she said, "I know you feel like your joy is gone forever, but it's not. One of these days — and it's gonna be sooner than you think — God's gonna give you joy again in one of His smallest blessings. You may not be expecting it. But it'll be there. And you'll feel that joy. I promise."

I wasn't prepared to be joyful right then. I didn't care about joy. Couldn't even imagine that joy would ever be possible again, but she was my grandmother and I loved her and respected that she'd walked this road before me, so I thanked her — and time went on.

My husband Richard and I worked together at a small minor emergency clinic on the outskirts of San Antonio. One day, about six weeks after Betsie's death, we were driving to work early in the morning. As we rounded a curve on Loop 1604, there, in a field that had been green the day before, lay a solid carpet of deep purple-blue. Texas bluebonnets had sprung up overnight and covered the field from edge to edge. I laughed out loud. "Look! That wasn't there yesterday!"

Then it struck me. I felt *joy* and it was there in one of God's smallest blessings. Or, rather, in thousands and thousands of God's smallest blessings, all put together in one place just for me.

I know that whoever sowed those seeds wasn't thinking of me. But God was. And He knew my heart. He knew what I needed. I needed those bluebonnets. He knew I'd be driving down that road at just the right moment.

Did that mean that everything was all right again? Of course not. There were still many, many, difficult days, weeks, months ahead. But I had been given a glimpse of joy, and recognized that I could still feel it — if only for a few moments. That was a blessing.

I don't know what your small blessing will be, but I know it will be there. Allow yourself to feel it. Allow yourself to laugh. Find your joy. Allow yourself to see that there is still life ahead — life to embrace and cherish and look forward to, with joy.

Steps of Coping After a Loss

Caregivers focus all their energy on protecting and caring for their child. Where do they focus all that energy and compassion after their loss?

The answer is unique to each person. But a good place to start is with a prayer asking for the Lord's guidance: "Lord, please continue to heal and comfort our broken hearts, and to open new doors to help others."

So, how do we cope with the loss of those who die before we do? No matter the age, we're never fully prepared, and nothing makes sense during those dark days.

"I take one step forward and five back," a mom said.

Often our first response to death is childlike: We think, "He's gone forever!" Or "That's not fair! He's mine!"

Many adults relate to death in these terms. And many times, we reel from one extreme to the other in our responses:

Fight: "Just what on earth do you think You're doing, God!"

Flight: "I give up. I can't feel You, God."

These are normal reactions. However, there's also a third possible reaction. This one is not controlled by your emotions like the first two, but it's controlled by your will-your choice to trust the "engineer" with the rest of the journey. That reaction demands that we step back and remember the truth that exists beyond our own feelings. That truth is expressed in this verse: "Therefore we do not lose heart. Even though our outward man is perishing, yet the inward man is being renewed day by day. For our light affliction, which is but for a moment, is working for us a far more exceeding and eternal weight of glory, while we do not look at the things which are seen, but at the things which are not seen. For the things which are seen are temporary, but the things which are not seen are eternal" (2 Corinthians 4:16-18).

We can't have all the answers when we want them, but as we go through life day by day, many answers do appear. However, many times our actions must come before answers. Hold on to this truth. He's taken you through the first part of your life (the good ol' days), and He will be there for the rest of the journey (the new normal) — one step at a time.

Corrie ten Boom knew dark tunnels in her life — from concentration camps to speaking all over the world until her 80's. As she said, "When you go through a dark tunnel, don't throw away the ticket and jump off. Sit still and trust the engineer."

She knew that engineer intimately.

Wherever you are on the journey: recently thrust into the tunnel; constantly thrown against the walls; or exiting into the sunlight, *you can still choose to take the life God has given you, and, with passion and purpose, complete what He has sent you here on earth to do.*

The Thickest Darkness

Night falls, and flowers fold their petals. Even in the thickest darkness, the heavenly dew falls — and it *only falls when the sun has gone.* God is there in the thickest darkness of our lives to give us songs in the night — His refreshing dew in our lives.

At the turn of the century, "night" had fallen for most of Annie Johnson Flint's life. From a very young age, she suffered from rheumatoid arthritis that left her crippled and bedridden. To alleviate the pain, she rested and slept on soft pillows. Her body developed serious bed sores and finally she suffered the ravages of cancer. Yet her attitude through all the struggles with pain and confinement was that of submission, faith and trust in God to give her the grace and the strength she needed. With a pen pushed through bent and gnarled fingers and held by swollen joints she wrote her verses which provided comfort for herself, her friends, and now the world. One such poem (now also a song) was "He Giveth More Grace."

He giveth more grace when the burdens grow greater,
He sendeth more strength when the labors increase;
To added affliction He addeth His mercy,
To multiplied trials, His multiplied peace.

His love has no limit, His grace has no measure;
His power no boundary known unto men;
For out of His infinite riches in Jesus
He giveth and giveth and giveth again.

When we have exhausted our store of endurance,
When our strength has failed ere the day is half done,
When we reach the end of our hoarded resources,
Our Father's full giving is only begun.

∼ Annie Johnson Flint, 1866-1932

We do reach the end of our hoarded resources — over and over, and over again. Our Father's full giving has only begun. You are not alone.

For God so loved the world that He gave His only begotten Son,
that whoever believes in Him should not perish
but have everlasting life.
John 3:16

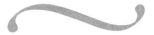

We've been given only one piece of life's jigsaw puzzle.
Only God has the cover of the box.

— Max Lucado

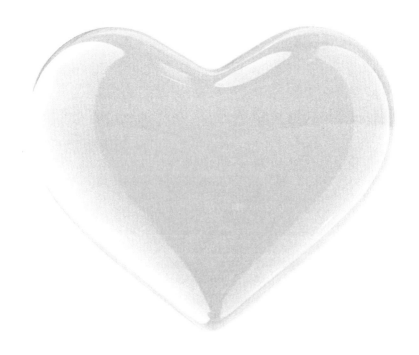

Afterwords

B eth picked up the blue and green curved puzzle piece and eyed the pieces she'd connected. *Where does this piece fit?* Each piece is only a small part of the completed picture. Some pieces along the edges are easier to place — they have at least one straight edge — and similar colors.

But then there are some puzzle pieces that don't seem to fit. Beth wedged that piece next to the curves of the other pieces. *It's got to fit somewhere.*

Some pieces of Beth's life fit easily — straight edges, predictable, comfortable, normal. Now she's stumped, this part (piece) of her life didn't fit, make sense, and wasn't comfortable. Beth's daughter Meghan faced more surgeries, and struggled as procedures, ports, feeding tubes, NG tubes, and "rolling" veins defied the IV sticks.

The picture Beth envisioned at the beginning of Meghan's life three years ago now has more misplaced pieces than ones that fit a "normal" picture.

Beth leaned over the table and studied the various colors and shapes. Did a piece get lost? *It doesn't make sense.*

Helps & Hope

Circumstances may appear to wreck our lives and God's plans, but God is not helpless among the ruins.
— Eric Liddell, Olympian

Some pieces of our life slip together easily; some take time and coaxing to fit. Others seemed to have slipped off the table. *Were some pieces lost at the manufacturer?*

Only the manufacturer has the cover of the box and knows where each piece fits. Paul in the New Testament had strewn pieces of his life—and by the world's standards; they would never be found or used. Here are Paul's words and perspective in I Corinthians 13:12, "For now we see in a mirror, dimly, but then face to face. Now I know in part, but then I shall know just as I also am known."

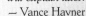

Helps & Hope

We are known by Him. "We do not serve a distant god who spouts encouraging clichés from the sideline. Instead, he enters into our suffering...God will never leave us on our own." Rick Warren, *The Purpose Driven Life: What on Earth Am I Here For?*

God writes across some of our days, will explain later.
— Vance Havner

You are not alone!

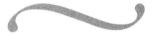

Resources

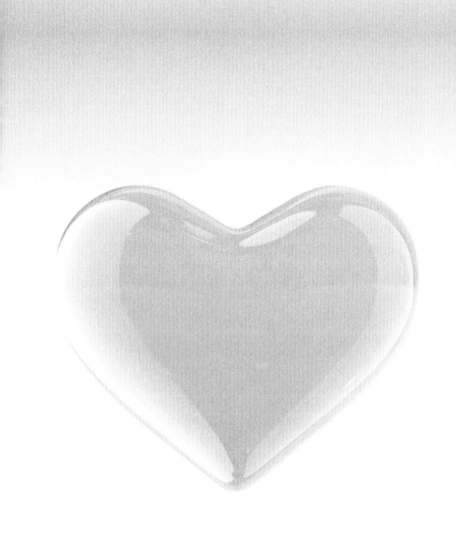

You-niquely Made

U sing the *You-niquely Made Personality Study* can help you understand and appreciate family, friends, and medical staff — all uniquely made. Jot notes to jog your memory of how to best meet their needs — and your needs also.

Vibrant Yellow's sunshine can brighten your day, but too much can drain you dry.

Sensitive Blue's rain clouds create beauty, but too many can be depressing.

Determined Red's instructions are helpful, but can be overbearing.

Calm Green's steadfast roots grow deep, but can be unmovable.

This resource should help you see the bright side of each color's personality and deal with each color's frailties.

Remember that each color and combination (blend) has strengths and weaknesses. Some move, eat, and speak slowly; some fast. Some need people around constantly; others want to be alone. To some, everything is either right or wrong; others go with the flow.

Each color has different coping skills.

The Yellow parent hits the wall but bounces back quickly and says, "Don't be so negative."

The opposite Blue parent wants all the information given correctly, and makes decisions slowly and thoroughly. "You can't make that decision off the top of your head," she says.

The Red parent doesn't want details, rabbit trails, or an idea that fails. "We're going to beat this!"

The opposite Green parent goes with the flow (as much as possible), listens, and when pressed to give an opinion, says, "Whatever they think best."

Different factors drain and fill their emotional tanks. Developing appreciation for each gene color will improve your communication and relationships. Appreciation prevents you from taking anyone for granted. God designed us to communicate effectively with others and with Him. He gave us His Designer genes.

King David said, "For You formed my inward parts; You covered me in my mother's womb. I will praise You, for I am fearfully and wonderfully made; Marvelous are Your works, And *that* my soul knows very well" (Psalm 139:13-14).

Vibrant Yellows

You hear Yellows before you see them — and continue to hear them, and hear them, and hear them. High energy, they bounce into rooms, eyes sparkling, wearing a perpetual smile. They pounce and hug anyone in reach. They make Tigger look passive.

To a Yellow, everyone is a best friend. They make those friends in elevators, standing in line at the grocery store, or answering a telemarketer's questions. Seldom wanting to be alone, they need "people fixes" often. Yellows begin many things, but they finish few. They constantly hear the following refrains:

✶ "How can you live in all that clutter?"

✶ "Where are your keys?"

✻ "You got lost where? Again?"

What drains their emotional tanks? Being alone and having to finish anything carefully (not simply slapping it together).

How do they react when their emotional tanks register empty? They talk more and louder. (Their opposites — the Blues can't imagine that Yellows can talk *more* or *louder*). If that doesn't work, they get totally quiet, and everyone says, "What's wrong with her, she's so quiet?"

How do you fill Yellow's emotional tank? You fill it with people — giving them time, talk, and touch (many hugs). You can also help them with organization.

So, how do Yellows fill others' tanks? They brighten a room.

We can all use the warmth they give, especially on dreary days.

Snapshot: When Yellow Brightened a Dreary Day

As Diane walked wearily from the parking garage to the hospital, her mind was preoccupied with her daughter's serious surgery.

"Well, hi there!" a tiny voice interrupted.

She looked around, then down. There stood a small, smiling boy. His father stood behind him, locking the car.

"Hi there," Diane replied.

"Whatchyoo doin' here?"

"I'm visiting my daughter. She's sick."

"I'm gonna see my nana," the boy said and rapidly shot the details.

His father sighed and said, "Son, leave the lady alone."

"Oh, that's okay."

The boy continued his story, as the father repeated, "Son, leave the lady alone."

To please the dad, Diane said, "I need to get on in. You have a good day." A few seconds later Diane was approaching the hospital door.

"Well, hi there," she heard the same boy say to a lady getting out of her car. "Whatchyoo doin' here?"

"Son, leave the lady alone."

Inside the hospital, as she headed down the gray corridor,

Diane smiled. "Thank You, Lord. I really needed that little ray of sunshine."

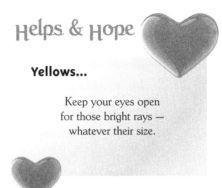

Helps & Hope

Yellows...

Keep your eyes open for those bright rays — whatever their size.

Helpful Hints if You're a Yellow

Yellows have trouble focusing — especially on things they don't want to do. Result? Things pile up and they feel overwhelmed. Yellows, focus on the first and most important task you need to do. Finish that before you go to the second. To do that, you may need to take small bites of the elephant. The task you've been putting off may look like an elephant, so remember this: you can't eat an elephant at one sitting. In the same way, you can't complete a huge task quickly. You have to take small bites — tackle small parts of the job. Here's a helpful hint: if you find you can't stay at a task for a long time. Set a timer for fifteen minutes. You can do almost anything for that length of time.

Take small bites; do parts of a big task, and be thankful for what you accomplish. Now what's that task you've put off? Cleaning a bathroom floor covered with dirty clothes and wet towels? Filing hospital papers and overdue bills? Finding your keys — again? Get started — not after one more computer game, telephone call, or e-mail excuse.

If you're a Yellow, you have to take the time to make a home for everything. Once you accomplish that task and put things back in their place, each time, it will become a habit. You'll put the dirty clothes and towels in the hamper, the mail in a certain stack (a shoebox will work), and the keys back on the hook. Surprisingly, you'll be able to find items when you need them and save valuable time and frustration. Blues do all of this instinctively.

Give Thanks for Yellows

Who are the Yellows in your life? Jot down their names and tell them thanks — they'll probably do even more. Even weary Yellows spread sunshine. Here are a few things to be thankful for in the Yellows you know:

* ✻ Continual contagious smile

* ✻ Hugs

* ✻ Friendliness — especially important to others who may be shy

* ✻ High energy level when others are winding down

* ✻ Click with children

Be thankful for those lights shining in the darkness.

Sensitive Blues

You've met the high-energy, talkative, outgoing Yellows. They multitask, start many projects, and finish few. Although their roller-coaster emotions zoom from tears to laughter, they still "go with the flow" as situations change. They see their glass at least half-full or overflowing as they spread their optimistic sunshine. Who are the Blues? In contrast to the Yellows, they're low-energy, quiet introverts. They do one thing at a time, slowly, and stay with it until it's completed perfectly. Their emotions, accompanied by sighing, register on two levels — deep and deeper. Blues don't like to go with the flow because transitions are traumatic. They need time to process the changes, and the new heart journey is packed with overwhelming transitions.

They see their glass half-empty — and draining. "Our half-empty glass is how the world really is," said a Blue. "At least we see things in an objective way."

We need Blue's devotion to detail, to jobs done well — such as balancing the checkbook to the penny — even if it takes them hours to do so. (Yellows guesstimate with checkbooks.) Blues correctly fill out hospital papers and meticulously place them in folders. Blues seriously think through situations, ponder, and in time give you their answer. People turn to them because they know Blues genuinely care. They read people well, but sometimes read into situations more than is there. When overwhelmed in a crisis, pushed to hurry up, or deprived of time alone, their emotional tank empties rapidly. They may become worn out or depressed, or they may simply shut down. As things build inside, an explosion may eventually erupt, leaving people confused. "What's wrong with her? She never acts like that, she's usually so quiet." If you're a Blue, you need to share what's going on. Let people know how you feel. No one can read your mind. How do you fill Blue's emotional tank? Give them lots of solitary time in a space of their own — away from crowds and noise — so they can process information. They live by their own time schedule and their way of doing things. Since transitions are traumatic, alert them to coming changes and give them time to adjust.

Who usually marry each other? Many times, it is opposite Yellows and Blues. Notice the totally different needs in Yellows and Blues? What helps one probably won't help the other; communication is desperately needed. While going through the tunnel, we especially need Blue's sympathy, hugs, and organizational skills.

Snapshot: Blue to the Rescue

"How's your wife doing?" Yellow Roy's voice boomed across the room.

"I got her home from the hospital Wednesday," the weary husband answered.

Roy slapped him on the back. "Well, that's great," he said while looking around the room.

The husband continued, "But I'm not sure where we go from here — "

"Uh huh," Roy replied as he spotted his next encounter and headed off, adding his traditional, "I'll be praying for you."

That's the picture. Yellow playing Duck, Duck, Goose, touching people as he continued in circles, not recognizing the deep need standing before him.

Then up walked Blue Dave, slipping his arm around the weary husband's shoulder.

"Claude, how's Jenny doing?"

As Claude related the last week's journey and the uncertainty of the tomorrows, Dave listened. He made Claude feel as if he were the only person in the room.

"I'm so sorry you're going through this. May I come by this afternoon and we'll talk?"

Noticing Claude's eyes brim with tears, Dave continued, "Can I pray with you right now?"

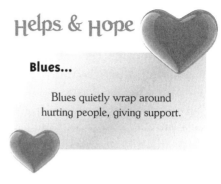

Helps & Hope

Blues...

Blues quietly wrap around hurting people, giving support.

Helpful Hints if You're a Blue

Life is a process not perfection. Your halfway effort will be better than almost everyone else's best tries, so don't procrastinate because you feel you have to attempt perfection.

Appreciate all that the different colors have to offer. You have deep feelings for others and take on their hurts, especially on this difficult journey. However, you may feel that optimistic Yellows aren't serious enough, driven Reds don't care enough, and passive Greens don't show enough emotion.

Pray for acceptance and appreciation of others. We're all in this together and desperately need each other.

Give Thanks for Blues

Who are they in your life? Jot down names and tell them thanks. They will appreciate your thoughtfulness. Here are a few things to be thankful for in the Blues you know:

* Feel deeply

* Support friends no matter what

* Organize everything

* Manage money (this journey needs that quality)

* Analyze decisions carefully

Be thankful for sensitive Blue genes.

Determined Reds!

Fasten your seatbelt — here come the Reds. They know what needs to be done, how to do it, and want it done now. They demand the bottom line (of whatever is happening) and don't care about details. Just get it done, then move on to the next task. Reds persevere no matter the obstacles and can't understand why everyone else doesn't do the same.

"I walked around on a broken leg for a week, she's complaining about a sprained ankle," stated a Red.

Two Reds together? They both think they're right. In a faceoff, they wait for the other to realize it.

"You should have seen the standoff between my child and her first doctor. I wasn't sure which one would win. It changed from day to day," said a mom.

They keep people's feet to the fire, not cutting them slack while working circles around everyone. So do they need their emotional tanks filled? Yes, whether they realize it or not. You can tell when they're on empty; they get louder and more demanding. If that doesn't work, they get totally quiet — everyone then waits for the other shoe to drop.

How do you fill a Red's tank? Give them appreciation for what they do — that's how they show love. Saying something like "Thanks for all your hard work getting this information and getting the job done" is music to their ears. Also, don't give them details, stay off rabbit trails, and simply give the bottom line.

When the going gets rough, you need a Red. Or if you simply need a guide.

Snapshot: A Trip to NYC

At a NYC hotel, a Red mom unpacked suitcases and said to her husband and daughter (both Blue-Greens), "I've made an agenda so we can make the best use of our time."

Dad and daughter smiled and rolled their eyes at each other.

"Mom, can I just rest for a few minutes?" moaned the teenager.

"We don't want to waste this weekend in the room."

"Do we have to walk everywhere?"

"Of course not. The subway's right across the street. Let's go."

The three headed out, agenda clutched in mom's hand. She walked briskly and spoke into the air, "Isn't this great!" Her husband and daughter knew the answer they were to give but were busy trying to keep up the pace. They raced down steep stairs leading to the subway. Mom stopped to check the subway map.

"Why do you want to look at this? You've got it all planned out," said her husband.

"It's fun to see where we are on the map and where we're going." She traced her finger along the color-coded routes. "Let's try this other line and see if we can cut off some stops."

"Mom, we're gonna get lost."

"Of course we won't. Besides, this is an adventure."

"Does the adventure include going back to the room this afternoon?"

"You really want to do that?"

"Can't I just rest for a little while?"

"OK, but you'll miss all the afternoon — "

"That's okay, Mom."

Backtracking to the hotel, daughter was left to rest and read. She was happy.

Mom hit the pavement in full stride, checking off her list. She was happy.

Dad attempted keeping up with mom. We think he was happy, but we know he was exhausted.

Back home, two days later, mom announced, "Wasn't that a great trip!"

"Uh huh," they answered.

Two months later, dad and daughter looked through the trip pictures again, "You know, that was fun," said dad.

"Yeah, but don't tell Mom."

Both smiled and rolled their eyes.

Helpful Hints if You're a Red

Stop, look, and listen:

Stop — or at least slow down. You're used to telling others to stop, now do so yourself.

Look — at others in the eye, not above their shoulder or at your watch.

Listen — to what others say.

Keep your opinions (how they could do things better) to yourself, unless asked. When you do speak the truth, do it in love. Be tactfully truthful.

Give your time, attention, and encouragement as gifts to others.

Helps & Hope

Reds...

Reds organize, prioritize, and best yet, they persevere. That's especially needed in tunnels.

They respect your opinion, especially if you've done the previous three steps.

Give Thanks for Reds

Who are they in your life? Jot down names and tell them thanks — if you can catch them. Here are a few things to be thankful for in the Reds you know:

∗ High energy, when others wind down

∗ Objectively see the big picture — what needs to be done and how to do it — give the bottom line

∗ Tenaciously persevere until a task is completed

∗ Keep self and others on task (hold their feet to the fire)

∗ Excel in a crisis ("He lives for times like this," is usually said of a Red)

Be thankful for those who shout, "Stop. I can help."

Calm Greens

Now sit back and relax. Can you hear the soothing sound of a porch swing clicking back and forth and back and forth and... That's like the go-with-the-flow, predictable Greens. Emotionally, they have no highs and no lows. They're great in a crisis. They get along with almost everyone. Greens go through life in slow motion — whether walking, talking, or eating. This pace drives Reds crazy. "When I tell her to hurry, she slows down!"

Reds and Greens are two more opposites who may end up marrying each other.

Greens don't demand attention so they can be easily overlooked. Of growing up in a household with more demanding siblings, a Green once said, "I felt invisible at the dinner table with my two brothers who hogged all the attention."

Teachers may not remember the names of their Green students because they're busy keeping up with the Reds and Yellows bouncing around the room.

Green's emotional tank drains slowly, but it does drain — especially when alone time becomes packed with people and activities. They become quieter, finally digging in their heels, not budging. Since they've gone along with everyone before, people are surprised at this reaction. "I told him we're going out to dinner, and he just sat there reading the paper. He wouldn't move!" stated a Red wife.

How do you fill these easygoing emotional tanks?

"You mean he really needs something?" asked his wife.

Yes, and since Greens don't demand attention, hearing their name or appreciation for what they've done will fill their tanks quickly. Remember their low energy level; they live for a good nap. Let them have one.

Greens are low-key, undemanding children who passively enter a low-key, undemanding adulthood.

Snapshot: Teacher's Lounge, 1984

"I'm so relieved they didn't laugh him off the stage." My teacher colleague was telling us about the speaker at her son's Ivy League college graduation that past weekend. "I watched as he sauntered up to the podium, smiled at the graduating class, and then he started singing: 'It's a beautiful day in the neighborhood....'

"I held my breath, as those unresponsive seniors stared silently at the stage. Then, during the song, they slowly melted into swaying three-year-olds leaning forward on their folding chairs. They even joined in singing his song. He had them in the palm of his hand. I can't remember what all he said, just how he said it. Then as he closed, they jumped to their feet clapping, whistling, and the girls rushed the stage shoving programs for his autograph. They yelled, 'Remember, me?' I guess they thought he'd seen them through the TV set years ago." All of us smiled and nodded as she continued.

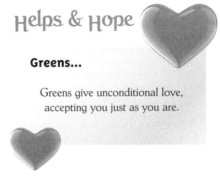

Helps & Hope

Greens...

Greens give unconditional love, accepting you just as you are.

"And, I loved all those sophisticated seniors shouting, 'Get my picture with my best friend, Mr. Rogers.' He just patiently stood there smiling with those kids as flashbulbs kept going off."

As a young child, extremely shy Fred Rogers was encouraged by his Grandfather McFeely. Fred became the nationally famous Mr. Rogers — encouraging generations through unconditional love.

Helpful Hints if You're a Green

Procrastination may be a familiar problem to you. Yellows procrastinate because they take on too much; Greens procrastinate because they use lack of energy as their excuse. Like Yellows, you need to take small bites of the elephant (see the helpful hints for Yellows). Greens need to focus, especially to finish tasks. You should also speak up and give feedback. Don't be prideful saying, "Hmm..., no one knows what I'm thinking." It's counterproductive. Also, others need your input to help make decisions. You have a balanced outlook. Yes, even Reds need it.

Give Thanks for Greens

Who are they in your life? Jot down names and be sure to thank them — by name. Here are a few things to be thankful for in the Greens you know:

∗ Sit and listen, don't interrupt

∗ Go with the flow; act rather than react

* Create calmness in crisis

* Reliable

* See things objectively

Be thankful for relaxed Green genes.

Ways We Give and Receive Love

Dovetailing with color-coded personalities is the understanding of how others give and receive love, Gary Chapman explains in his book *The Five Love Languages: Ways You Give and Receive Love.* Who needs what in your family to refill those empty emotional tanks?

According to Chapman's book, love is given and received in five primary languages:

* Talk — "Let me hear something positive. I need to know I'm doing something right."

* Touch — Babies thrive on it; children feel special with it; teens may not acknowledge it, but desire a passing nudge; adults sometimes admit, "I just need a hug."

* Time — "Just sit down and spend time with me. Don't be glancing at your watch."

* Gifts — "I can't believe my sister gave me a little shell from last summer's trip. And you know, gifts don't have to cost anything — just that someone thinks about you in a tangible way. Also, I can glance at the shell and relive the moment for a long time."

* Deeds — "OK, so you say, 'I love you,' a lot. When you pick your wet towels off the floor and hang them up, I'll know you mean it. Actions speak louder than words."

"My wife 'speaks' three of the love languages, and I speak the other two. Amazing we communicate at all," a husband said and laughed.

Which languages are important to you? How about others in your family? Talk it over and each week have everyone write down one thing they need. As the family meets each other's emotional needs, everyone wins. Pray for the willingness and follow-through to give these gifts — in and out of the tunnel.

Chapman's books have strengthened families and influenced countless relationships. More information on his books is given in Resource Two.

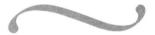

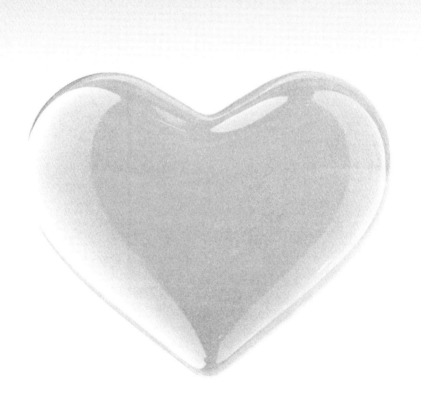

Inspirational Reading List

Gary Chapman's books on Love Languages gives insights into ways we can "speak" encouragement to each other — with words, quality time, giving gifts, acts of service, and touch.

Gary Chapman and Ross Campbell, *The Five Love Languages of Children* (Northfield Press, 2005).

Gary Chapman, *The Five Love Languages of Teens* (Northfield Press, 2005).Gary Chapman, *The Five Love Languages: How to Express Heartfelt Commitment to Your Mate* (Northfield Press, 2004).

Gary Chapman, *The Five Love Languages of God* (Northfield Publishing, 2002).

John R. Claypool, *Tracks of a Fellow Struggler: Living and Grieving Through Grief* (Morehouse Pub Co, 2003).

Nancy Guthrie, *The One Year Book of Hope* (Tyndale House, 2005).

Two of Carol Kent's books share this speaker-author's shattered life, and how God rebuilt the pieces on her journey. Carol knows what it means to live with an unthinkable circumstance that will never change — and to still make hope-filled choices.

Carol Kent, *A New Kind of Normal, Hope-Filled Choices When Life Turns Upside-Down* (Thomas Nelson, 2007).

Carol Kent, *When I Lay My Isaac Down: Unshakable Faith in Unthinkable Circumstances* (Navpress, 2004).

Ann Graham Lotz, *Why? Trusting God When You don't Understand* (Thomas Nelson, 2005).

Max Lucado, *God Came Near* (Thomas Nelson, 2004).

Robert J. Morgan, *Red Sea Rules: The Same God Who Led You in Will Lead You Out* (Thomas Nelson, 2001).

Barbara Robinson, *Best Christmas Pageant Ever* (HarpCollins, 1972).

Philip Yancey, *Prayer: Does It Make Any Difference?* (Zondervan, 2006).

Philip Yancey, *Reaching for the Invisible God, what can we expect to find?* (Zondervan, 2000).

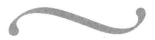

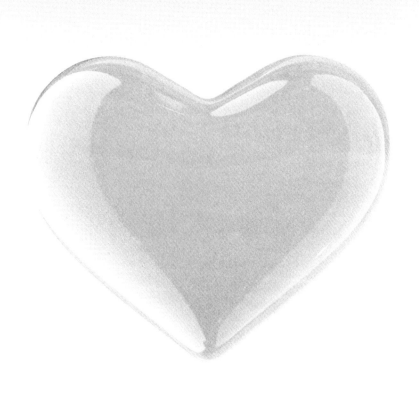

Resource Three

Organizations
and Websites

Organizations & Websites

The following associations and organizations are helpful sources of additional information for your journey.

American Heart Association (AHA)
www.americanheart.org
The American Heart Association provides material on congenital heart defects, types of medical treatment / testing, a glossary of terms and other helpful information.

The Children's Heart Foundation (CHF)
www.childrensheartfoundation.org
The Children's Heart Foundation (CHF) - funds the most promising research to advance the diagnosis, treatment and prevention of congenital heart defects.

Congenital Heart Defects

www.congenitalheartdefects.com
Whether you are looking for definitions of medical terms, hospitals caring for people with CHDs, other people with whom you can network and share experiences, links to support groups, articles regarding CHDs, or resources for the CHD community, you have come to the right place! Congenital Heart Defects website sponsored by Baby's Heart Press.

CareFlash

www.careflash.com
Free personal websites for patients and families involved in medical circumstances. 3-D animations and related medical links also.

Carepages

www.carepages.com
Free, personal, and private web pages that help family and friends communicate when someone is receiving care.

Caringbridge

www.caringbridge.org
Offers free, easy-to-create websites that help connect friends and family when they need it most.

Hearts of Hope SE Michigan

www.heartsofhopemi.org
Non-profit organization located in the Metro Detroit area. Our mission is to provide support, hope, resources, and networking to families affected by congenital heart defects. We offer parent-matching, on-line support groups, newsletters, and annual events for heart families.

It's My Heart

www.itsmyheart.org
Its mission is to provide support, spread awareness, educate and advocate for those affected by Acquired and Congenital Heart Defects by creating alliances with fellow families, hospitals, support groups, and the community.

Kids With Heart: National Association for Children's Heart Disorders

www.kidswithheart.org

Our organization was formed in 1985 with the main mission of providing support, information, and education for the families of the children living with congenital heart defects and to promote public awareness of the issues that these families live with on a day to day basis.

Little Hearts, Inc.

www.LittleHearts.net, www.littlehearts.org

A non-profit organization founded in January 1998. We provide support, resources, networking, and hope to families affected by congenital heart defects. Membership consists of families nationwide who have or are expecting a child with a congenital heart defect.

March of dimes

www.modimes.com

The March of dimes provides information and much more on all birth defects including congenital heart defects.

Mended Little Hearts

www.mendedlittlehearts.org

Mended Little Hearts, a new support program for parents of children with heart defects and heart disease, is dedicated to inspiring hope in those who care for the littlest heart patients of all. Mended Little Hearts offers resources and a caring support network as families find answers and move forward to find healing and hope.

Helping Hands Healing Hearts

www.riheartgroup.com

Helping Hands Healing Hearts is a support group for RI and Eastern Mass. For families of children with CHD. It is a chapter of Mended Little Hearts.

Ronald McDonald House Charities

www.rmhc.com

Many major cities have these facilities where out-of-town families can stay while their children are being treated for a serious illness. Room rates are economical, and a social worker may be able to help locate one.

Saving Little Hearts
www.savinglittlehearts.org
Saving Little Hearts has been helping children with congenital heart defects and their families since 2002. This organization is dedicated to helping children with congenital heart defects and their families by providing financial and emotional assistance and educational information. Saving Little Hearts also strives to provide enriching, educational and fun experiences for these children which will help them build friendships and confidence.

Songs of Love
www.songsoflove.org
The Songs of Love Foundation is an nonprofit organization dedicated to providing personalized songs for chronically ill children and young adults. These one of a kind compositions are a wonderful source of joy and inspiration to the special people who receive them. Visit their site and request a song for your child today. Just click on the "Request a Song" link, fill out the form, send it in, and within weeks, your child will be able to listen to his/her unique song

The Congenital Heart Information Network (TCHIN)
www.tchin.org
The Congenital Heart Information Network (TCHIN) ~ provides reliable CHD information, resources, internet links, as well as support for families, adults, and health professionals.

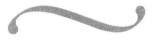

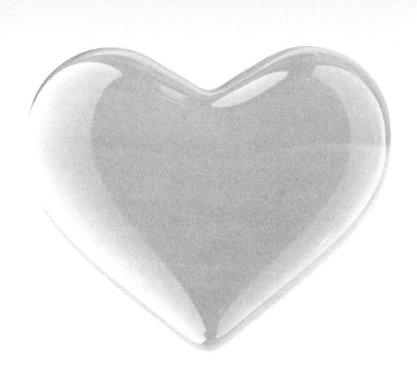

Resource Four

Scriptural Index

God's love
1 John 4:19, p.80
Mark 10:13-16, p.44

God's plans for you (here on earth)
Jeremiah 29:11, p.21
Galatians 5:14, p.117
2 Corinthians 5:7, p.131
Psalm 139:13-14, p.152

God's plans for you (for future life)
John 3:16, p.143
I Corinthians 13:12, p.146

God's rest
Matthew 11:28, p.5
Psalm 23:1-2, p.57

God's strength
Ephesians 6:10, p.45
Deuteronomy 33: 22-23, p.56
2 Corinthians 12:9, p.68
2 Timothy 4:17, p.67
Psalm 73:26, p.85
Psalm 28:7, p.83
2 Corinthians 4:8-9, p.137
2 Corinthians 4:16-18, p.141

Peace
Isaiah 26:3, p.77
Psalm 46:10, p.81
Philippians 4:7, p.109

Prayer
Philippians 4:6, p.97

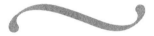

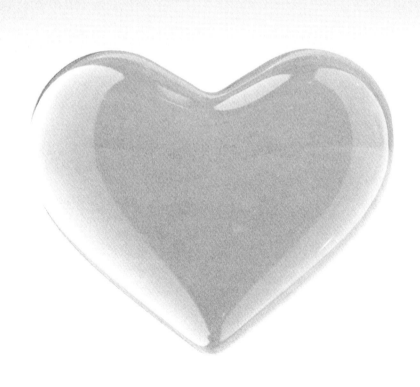

About the Author

Lynda Young is co-founder of *Kindred Spirits International*. Through conferences, books, publications, and ministries, KSI outreaches include children's hospitals, women's groups, medical community, and Amani ya Juu, refugee women's mission in Nairobi, Kenya.

A member of American Association of Christian Counselors, Lynda is a nationwide speaker, award-winning author/writer. She continually shares her passion for helping others 'come along-side' families who are hurting when their children are suffering.

She holds masters degrees in Religious Education from Southwestern Baptist Theological Seminary and Education/Administration from University North Carolina. Her work includes positions as a teacher/administrator, and has published and taught *You-niquely*

Made© curricula on personalities. She holds memberships in American Christian Writers, Christian Writers Fellowship International, and Advanced Writers and Speakers Association. She is also a graduate of Speak Up with Confidence and CLASSeminars.

Lynda's first book in the "You Are Not Alone" book series, *Hope for Families of Children with Cancer,* won the Living Now Silver Book Award: Parenting category. Lynda continues her writing in this series with more books for parents of children with chronic conditions.

Lynda and her husband John have four children, eleven grandchildren, and three great-grandchildren — lots of hands on experience. Her husband, Dr. John L. Young, has been in Cancer Research Statistics on a national and international level since 1965, and is a professor at Emory University. They live in Snellville, GA (suburb of Atlanta) and are active at Annistown Road Baptist Church. Lynda Tinnin Young grew up in Oklahoma City, where her father, Rev. Finley Tinnin was pastor at Baptist Temple.

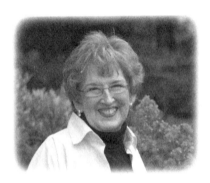

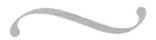

You Are Not Alone!
Lynda Young Shares with Parents, Families, Caregivers

Lynda Young speaks from her heart and touches thousands with her clear message that *You Are Not Alone!* With energy, passion and extensive experience, she travels the journey with families, caregivers and caring friends of children who are hurting.

Lynda brings hope and calm in the midst of distress and suffering. Come along with Lynda as she brings clarity of what IS possible during the journey and how to actively contribute in new ways that brings comfort to all involved. Her topics include...

♥ *I'm Sorry to Tell You This, Your Child Has ...*
Journeying along with families who hear the news, and need to understand and cope with the 'new normal'

♥ **When Your Emotional Tank Registers Empty**
Effective communication tools during stressful situations

♥ **Siblings: the Invisible Ones**
Meeting the needs of the "well" one

♥ **"Root wrapping"**
Strengthening others during a crisis — helping the hurting

Bring Lynda Young to your church groups, retreats,
and conferences to speak with parents, families, caregivers,
church leadership, Stephens Ministries and counselors.

For more information visit
www.HopeForFamiliesOnline.com or
www.LyndaYoung.com